HOW'S YOUR MOM?

WHAT YOU REALLY WANT TO SAY WHEN YOUR MOM HAS MS

A MEMOIR

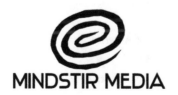

MINDSTIR MEDIA

How's Your Mom?
What you really want to say when your mom has MS

Published by Mindstir Media, LLC
45 Lafayette Rd | Suite 181| North Hampton, NH 03862 | USA
1.800.767.0531 | www.mindstirmedia.com

Printed in the United States of America
ISBN-13: 978-1-7327049-3-0
Library of Congress Control Number: 2018909850

HOW'S YOUR MOM?

WHAT YOU REALLY WANT TO SAY WHEN YOUR MOM HAS MS

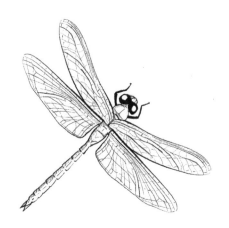

A MEMOIR

MICHELLE LEBS
WITH TAMRA DEVINE

DEDICATION

For my mom and dad.
Thank you for painting the greatest portrait of love that I have
ever seen, and for including me in it.
I love you.

DISCLAIMER

Each case of multiple sclerosis presents itself differently, and this story is mine and mine alone. It is not meant to reflect every individual's experience. This book is not intended as a substitute for the medical advice of physicians. The reader should consult with a physician in matters relating to his/her health. All characters, incidents, and dialogue are real, but some of the names and identifying details in this book have been changed to protect the privacy of individuals.

FOREWORD

TAMMY

In general, I didn't want to die. I didn't think about death. I didn't even wonder about it. I didn't have a bucket list, and I didn't live my life to the fullest because each day could have been my last. I was neither prophetic nor profound enough to engulf myself in that much virtuosity.

When my kids were little, we would take a plane ride in February to visit my parents who were snowbirds in Florida. Here I was, this not-so-seasoned adventurist with a preschooler and second-grader in tow. Yeah, it did occur to me that I should have a plan in case of emergency. I contemplated *Sophie's Choice*, but that was just too upsetting. So instead I told my kids a little story.

"If the plane should happen to get into trouble, and if we are crashing, this is what you do," I said calmly, seriously. I ran my fingers through Alex's wavy blond hair, took a deep breath and looked into his sparkling blue eyes. I turned to Michelle and smoothed down her angel-soft blonde hair, wishing she could stay this small forever. Their tiny faces stared back at me, eager to hear the answer of how their mommy would keep them safe in any circumstance. I took a deep breath. "You put your head between your legs . . . and you kiss your ass good-bye."

They stared blankly at me, then at each other. Alex smiled, although only seven years old, he already understood my sarcastic sense of humor. Michelle didn't quite get it, but she copied whatever her older brother did. The three of us sat there smiling while I double-checked their seat belts. It was truly the best advice I could give!

My husband, Chris, and I loved to take day trips together but I was always a homebody and never liked leaving home for more than a few days. Occasionally, we would drive his 1970 Chevelle an hour west to the farms of New Hampshire or an hour south to the ocean in Massachusetts.

One beautiful summer day, we had nothing better to do.

"Let's take a drive!" Chris exclaimed at seven that morning.

What the hell? I thought. *Why not?*

We drove to the coast of Massachusetts, then lunched at Scituate Harbor. We took pictures of Scituate Lighthouse, and then we drove through Brant Rock. Chris turned into an open parking lot facing the water and turned off the engine, then opened all the windows. I closed my eyes, listened to the ocean sounds and breathed in the salty air. *Ah, the simple things in life.*

Lest you think I am the only family member with a warped sense of humor, Chris interrupted my relaxing thoughts with his query, "What would you do if a huge wave suddenly rose out of the ocean and came over the sea wall?" I chuckled. I thought to myself, *I have MS, you know. That is what happens to me every day.* But I told him what I knew he wanted to hear.

"I'd put my head between my legs and kiss my ass good-bye."

So, I didn't sit around contemplating death. I didn't even contemplate life. I was just there for the ride, thinking about the eternal question that humanity loves to meditate on: *Is it about the goal or the journey?* Either way, I thought that when all was said and done, I would simply put my head between my legs and kiss my ass good-bye, like I had told my kids to do. But when push finally did come to shove, I couldn't just give in like I had planned.

I didn't know that I possessed the strength to hold my head up high instead of burying it between my legs. But when I needed that strength, I found it. Or, maybe, *it* found *me.* Maybe that's just what happens when you get diagnosed with multiple sclerosis—you start uncovering all your secret superpowers.

*_*_*_*_*_*

And now, as I *always* say *sometimes*, all anyone really wants is to be remembered.

PART ONE
THE SEARCH
JULY 2007–NOVEMBER 2009

CHAPTER ONE

MICHELLE

Mom was trying to bend over when the crash happened, and it was completely my fault.

I was twenty-one years old, home for the summer after completing my junior year of college, and Mom and I were in the middle of baking banana bread. I had been listening closely to her directions. "Mix the dry ingredients first. You need one of these and one of these," she told me as she reached up from her seated position on her walker to the countertop and placed a teaspoon on the baking soda and a half-teaspoon on the salt. She had made the recipe so many times that she had the whole thing memorized.

For as long as I could remember, Mom made the world's best banana bread. She was an incredible baker, a skill she inherited from my grandmother, who we lovingly referred to as Bubbie. She could bake just about anything you asked her to, but banana bread was her claim to fame. It was so good that my best friend, Hannah, and I got into a serious argument about it in third grade, each strongly believing that her own mom made the better banana bread. In the end, we had to agree to disagree, or else forfeit our entire friendship.

Mom had shown me, in the time we would come to refer to as "before," as in *before multiple sclerosis came into our lives,* exactly how to measure dry ingredients. You needed to delicately fluff the flour as you scooped it into the measuring cup, then use the back of a knife to level it out perfectly across the top. Baking was a precise art. "You can't be as loosey-goosey as you can be when you cook," she had taught me. When you baked, you had to follow the recipe exactly.

Now, she sat solemnly with her shoulders hunched forward, looking tired and disengaged. She'd been diagnosed with MS two years before, in 2009. She was wearing a white tank top with a sports bra underneath, and stretchy, cotton, elastic-waist pants— the only clothes she could still take on and off by herself. She had showered that morning, and her short, curly hair was still damp. She was too exhausted to stand and help me. It was all she could do to give me verbal instructions while I gathered ingredients and assembled the recipe myself.

It was July 2011, and we were in the cozy kitchen of my family's home in New Hampshire, the place we'd called home since my parents purchased the house brand new in 1999. My parents fell in love with the house both for its location and layout. It was designed like a ranch, with all the rooms my parents would need located on the first floor, and only me and my older brother Alex's bedrooms on the second floor, as well as an additional bathroom. "It's going to be a great house to grow old in," Dad had told me when I asked him curiously, at nine years old, why we had to leave the much smaller place we already called home. Dad was planning for their future. He knew they would want to retire in a ranch.

It turned out to be a good thing they bought that house, because now, at fifty years old, Mom already needed a walker.

"Add a cup of whole wheat flour and a half cup of white flour," she told me, her personal modification for a healthy version. I did as I had been trained to do and added it to the bowl of dry ingredients.

"Now you want to start mixing the eggs. Go turn on the Kitchen Aid," she told me. Again, I did as I was told. "Next, go mash the bananas," she said, and although she didn't mean for it to sound like an order, that was how I heard it.

We liked to use a particular Pyrex measuring glass when we mashed the bananas because it made them easier to transfer into the Kitchen Aid when it was time to combine it all. The Pyrex glass lived in a cabinet under the island counter, behind where Mom had been sitting on her walker. I could have asked her to move and told her I would get it. But I wanted her to *do something*. She had just been sitting there, telling me what to do, ordering task after task. Baking banana bread was supposed to be something we were doing *together*. But this wasn't how normal mothers and daughters did things *together*. This was not enjoyable for me.

So, instead of getting it myself, like I could have, I asked her to get it. I knew this would mean she would have to stand, take a few steps to clear the cabinet door, open it, bend over, reach for the Pyrex dish and lift it onto the counter . . . but I wanted her to do it. I didn't care if she had MS, she needed to do *something* to help.

"Mom, can you get the Pyrex glass?" I asked.

Her face twisted in a momentary knot of uncertainty. "Sure," she told me, against what was clearly her better judgement.

Confidently, I turned my back on her and walked toward the Kitchen Aid on the opposite side of the kitchen. I added the softened butter, vanilla extract, applesauce (another healthy alternative) and half of the required amount of sugar to the two eggs already in the bowl and watched them all combine.

That's when she screamed my name.

"MICHELLE!" she bellowed with a scary, scratchy strain in her voice.

I was only about three steps away from her, but it didn't matter. I couldn't respond quickly enough. I couldn't move fast enough. I turned my head before moving my legs and watched her lose her balance and begin to fall.

I took one step, as her legs tangled beneath her, her arms still held tightly to the sides of her walker, momentarily frozen and ultimately useless.

I took another step as her knees crashed into the hardwood.

Another step . . . I was only one step away now . . . and her forearms and elbows hammered down, drilling themselves into the floor.

On the last step, I reached out to save the very last thing that was yet to hit the floor—her head. I reached both of my arms forward, extending them as long as I could, but they fell short.

I fell short.

Her head smashed angrily into the floor, her top lip scraping the corner of the cabinet the whole way down.

My knees melted into the floor as I frantically examined her seemingly lifeless body lying face down on the floor next to me. A pool of blood began to form on the floor next to her lip. I watched the tears begin to fall from her face and felt them fall from on my own as well.

I thought about all the things we should do at that moment: She should sit up. She should sit on her walker. She should get a Band-Aid. She should get ice. She needed a tissue. She needed a hug. She needed to lay still for a minute. What should she do? What should I do?

My mind raced with possibilities. But I couldn't do any of them. I was frozen.

Her sobs filled the house, and it was all I could to keep mine contained. I might have been crying, but I was certain that if I kept my mouth shut, I could pretend the tears weren't really there. That none of this was really happening.

Whether five seconds or five minutes passed, I had no idea. All I knew was that Dad appeared, instantly meeting Mom's gaze from ground level. "What happened, baby?" he cooed as he stroked her hair.

"She fell," I sputtered at him as my tears poured onto the floor, my silence finally broken. The act of admitting it out loud made my heart physically hurt.

"It's okay, Shell," he told me. We both struggled to take our eyes off of Mom. "Can you get her some ice?" Grateful for the direction, I nodded my head furiously, eager to escape the hideousness that had just unfolded in front of me.

As I stood and began to walk away, I heard Dad whisper phrases in her ear that I couldn't quite make out. He was still stroking her curly hair, tucking it neatly behind her ear, bringing her back to safety. That's what Dad always did best—he made us all feel safe.

I returned a moment later with boo-boo bear, the small, bear-shaped cotton washcloth that Mom used to tuck an ice cube into and give to Alex and me whenever we got hurt. The irony of giving her the same icepack now sent chills down my spine. It wasn't right.

Dad pressed it to her lip until she finally caught her breath, still lying face down on her stomach. When her tears stopped, and the world started turning again, Dad and I helped her to her feet and lifted her back into a sitting position on her walker. "Let's bring you to bed," Dad suggested. I watched Mom nod, then saw their backs turn away from me as Dad pushed her down the hallway and into their bedroom.

I turned back around and glanced around the kitchen. My gaze landed squarely on the Kitchen Aid, which was still obliviously mixing the wet ingredients. The wrapper from the butter and the container from the applesauce were lying scattered in a trail of flour on the counter. The loaf pan, already coated with nonstick cooking spray, sat empty on the stovetop. The dry ingredients waited patiently in their bowl.

I thought about leaving the entire mess there. If Mom couldn't help, I didn't want to do it. I wanted to quit like she had been forced to do. I shook my head, completely disappointed in my own stupid demand for Mom to help. Why hadn't I just pushed her walker aside and gotten the Pyrex glass myself?

It didn't matter what I did or didn't do. *The shoulda, woulda, couldas fix nothing,* I could hear Mom telling me in my head like she had so many times before. *All we can do is live and learn.*

As I stared hard at the mess in front of me, I thought about what she would have wanted me to do. She wouldn't have wanted me to quit. She had taught me to always keep going when things got hard. I knew she was going to want a piece of the banana bread tonight.

Feeling like a robot, and nothing like myself, I pulled out the Pyrex glass from the cabinet, and carried on, assembling the entire banana bread on my own, hearing Mom's instructions in my head with each step. *Don't overmix the flour,* her voice echoed in my head as I added it to the mashed banana mixture.

Later that night, Dad, Alex, Mom, and I all ate slices of banana bread. It somehow turned out to be the best loaf I ever made. Dad thanked me as he loaded his empty plate into the dishwasher, then patted his hand on the top of my head.

"You're a good cook, Shell," he said. "You must have gotten that trait from your Bubbie. Thanks for makin' it."

I knew it wasn't much, but I was glad I'd finished making it.

I was glad I didn't give up.

CHAPTER TWO

TAMMY

I used to be a health nut and avid runner.

I didn't run to lose weight, although that was a nice perk. I just ran because I liked it. I started running when I was around forty years old. I hadn't told myself I was going to become a runner or even signed up for any races when I was first inspired to run. Instead, running seemed to fall literally into my path.

One summer evening, Michelle and I were out on one of our after-dinner walks around the neighborhood. She was around ten years old, and we both enjoyed taking walks together. It was our chance to chat privately, without the boys of the house listening in on us. As an added bonus, we could burn off some extra calories and feel less guilty about the bowl of ice cream we would eat when we got home. (Although I was a firm believer that if you ate ice cream straight from the carton while standing at the counter, the calories didn't count.)

"Michelle, let's see if we can run to that stop sign," I told her as I pointed to the sign about two telephone poles away from us. She didn't argue. We looked at each other, and then we were running!

Michelle's long legs swiftly carried her ahead of me. Her wavy blonde ponytail bounced along behind her, and she beat me to the stop sign. I met her there moments later, and we continued walking forward together. "Let's do it again!" I told her, pointing to the next one. We continued sprinting between stop signs and telephone poles, taking breaks to walk in between.

We must have run two miles that first night, and that was how running started for me. We went out a few more times together until Michelle grew bored with the idea. "Running isn't fun for me," she told me. "I don't want to go again, but you can still go." Although I was disheartened that she didn't want to accompany me anymore, I really wanted to run. So I went.

I continued going out every night for "walking runs," as I

called them, increasing the length of time I ran between each telephone pole a little more every day. It only took me a few weeks to work up the endurance to be able to run a three-mile loop around my neighborhood.

I was addicted to the sensation that I felt after a good run. Eventually, I started waking up early in the morning so I could run before work. Waking up at four thirty a.m. became a habit. I wasn't trying to lose weight, but I was. Plus, I could eat an extra cookie at night if I wanted to. The high I got lasted all morning and most of the afternoon. When I was at work, I would wait for the opportunity to be able to say, *Boy, it was a good day for a run.*

Truthfully, every day was a good day for a run. When I looked out the window and at the thermostat to see the temperature outside each morning, I wasn't looking to see if the conditions were conducive for a run. Rather, I was looking to see what I should wear. Sweatshirt or fleece jacket, shorts, capris, or long pants. Should I bring a hat and gloves? I always stuck a hanky in my sleeve or a pocket. When evening came, I started to think about the next morning's run. I solved all the world's problems during my runs. I told my boss off, and I planned my children's futures during my runs.

Before every run, Chris liked to jokingly ask, "Do you have your ID on ya? I want them to be able to identify the body if they find you lying in the street."

He was kidding, of course, but it still stuck in my head. As I sorted through the mail one day, I couldn't help my excitement when I saw the latest issue of *Runner's World.* I did a precursory flip through of the magazine and landed on a page with an advertisement for a tag that attached to your shoelaces. It was a small, shiny, silver disc that could be engraved with your choice of words or a picture. I chose the one that said, "I run because I can." I added my personal identification number to the flip side. The tag arrived in the mail days later, and I secured it firmly to my shoelaces. It accompanied me on every run.

I used to pray to G-d that he would never take my ability to run away from me.

After about a year of regular running, a postcard arrived in my mailbox from Team in Training, a nonprofit dedicated to raising money for myeloma and leukemia research. The group trained participants and taught them how to run a marathon. Although the postcard didn't have my name on it, it might as well have. I felt like it was destiny. My father-in-law had just passed away from multiple myeloma months before. I thought about it for only a few quick seconds before I picked up the phone and called my sister-in-law, Trudy, who was also a runner. "This is destiny," I told her. "We're going to do this for your dad."

Multiple locations hosted informational meetings for learning about the team. I attended a meeting at the Nashua Public Library, located a few miles from my house, and Trudy attended a meeting closer to hers in Massachusetts. The fact that I actually took myself there alone was a feat in itself. I was the type of person who didn't go anywhere alone. I was more of a buddy-system kind of person, but this was a lone adventure for me. The fact that I was doing it amazed me, yet I wouldn't have it any other way.

The meeting was short and sweet. It convinced me that I wanted to do this thing, so I signed up.

The training runs were so much fun for me. Again, that I was doing all this independently amazed me. I drove myself to the different places for the training runs and met some nice people. I met a wonderful friend named Karen, who ran at the exact same pace as I did. For that reason, she became my running buddy.

On the day of the marathon, Karen and I ran the entire way together. At one point, she left me to go relieve herself in a bush. I slowed down enough to let her do her thing and catch back up to me. As independent as I had been in taking myself to all the training runs, I didn't want to lose her on the marathon run.

The marathon got hard at mile twenty. My legs ached as I searched for the finish line. Leading up to it, I spied my good friend from college, Kathleen, on the sidelines with her daughter, Cara. Cara had leukemia when she was a little girl, but kicked its butt due to the life-saving effect of a bone marrow transplant she'd been given by a donor.

My Team in Training trainer met us just before the finish line and ran through it with us with our arms raised high in the air. We did it! We finished in four hours and twelve minutes.

I don't remember what my children's reaction was. I don't know if they felt my joy and sense of accomplishment. I don't know if they felt pride or if they were just glad it was over because now they would have their mom back to give them her full attention again.

But I didn't stop running after the marathon training ended. My morning runs weren't as necessary because I wasn't training for anything, but I still did them.

I ran until everything changed.

It started when I took a fall in July 2007. I was forty-six years old and had been a real *runner* for about six years by then. At first, I didn't think much of it. A coworker friend told me she had fallen more than a few times during her runs. She said she occasionally tripped over curbstones, so I blamed my first fall on a sewer cover. With the scratched cheek and a bruised shoulder, I felt I would wear my wounds proudly.

The next time I tripped, about a month later, I was actually at the same place in a run. I blamed that one on the fact that I'd glanced over my left shoulder to see a deer running across the street. I picked myself up and carried on that time. I got a tingly feeling in my left arm and tried to shake it off. I thought maybe it was because the arm stayed in a bent position for so long throughout the run.

A few weeks later, I started getting drop foot in my left foot. Drop foot made it very hard for me to lift the front part of my foot up off the ground. My foot felt instantly weak, and I didn't know why. I couldn't come up with any excuses for it. I would run through it and sang cadences like *"Lift your foot, don't let it drop, or you will fall and be real sad."* The run would go on. I made it to the end and did my stretches. I liked to hang down at my waist, hold on to my ankles, and look at the trees behind me while upside down. I felt like I was getting a new view of the world.

One morning, as I sat on my steps to cool down and

dropped my head, I felt an electric shock run down my neck. It made me pause, but I still didn't think anything of it.

I continued running for a few months. Occasionally, my vision wobbled. The horizon seemed to bounce. It reminded me of *The Blair Witch Project*. I'd never seen the movie, but I'd seen previews. There was someone running with a camcorder in the woods. As the videographer ran, everything kind of bounced around. That's what the world sometimes looked like to me.

On very rare occasions, with no warning, my body would just quit on me. I couldn't run anymore. It wasn't that I was tired. It felt like someone high above had reached down, pushed on my head, and made me stop. When that happened, I stopped running and tried to walk, dragging my feet underneath me. It felt like my driveway was a million miles away, even though it was only a few yards in front of me.

That was the end of running and the beginning of the search for answers.

CHAPTER THREE

MICHELLE

Mom's journey with multiple sclerosis began long before I had any clue what was happening. It was 2008, I was eighteen years old, and preparing to begin my adult life by heading off to college and moving out of my parents' house.

As a high school senior, I wasn't the kind of kid who was excited to move out of her parents' house, head off to college, forget my responsibilities, and party all night long. I wasn't interested in attending a college located across the country and putting as much distance between my parents and me as possible. I wasn't excited about the idea of having no curfew or being able to stay out as late as I pleased. Actually, my biggest concern was finding a college that would allow me to keep my parents just far enough away. If I extended my arms, I wanted to know I could reach them. But I didn't want to be so close that extending my arms would force me to bump into them, either.

Much to my surprise, I found myself falling in love with a small state school, Keene State College, about an hour away from my hometown in New Hampshire. Unlike Mom, who had been told by her parents that if she wanted them to pay for college, she had to go to a state school, I had been given the freedom to make my own decision. It didn't matter where I went, but I would be paying my way through no matter what. I thought I wanted to attend a real university, no matter how much it was going to cost. My parents cautioned me that attending an out-of-state, private university would mean I would have more student debt to pay off after graduation. Given the fact that I wanted to be a teacher, I knew I shouldn't graduate with a huge amount of debt. Nonetheless, a piece of me didn't care. I was pleasantly surprised to learn that I could love a small, affordable school just as much (if not more) than a large university.

In the summer leading up to my departure for school, Mom did her best to think of everything I might possibly need to feel comfortable in my new home-away-from-home. We filled our days with trips to Bed Bath and Beyond, Target, the mall, and Costco trying to ensure we purchased everything I might possibly need. She thought of everything: a shower caddy, posters for my walls, ink for my printer, rain boots, a cozy carpet, extra-long twin-sized bed sheets, granola bars, and sugar for my coffee. My "dorm room crap," as Alex, who was a senior at Bridgewater State College at the time, had called it, took up the entire living room all summer long.

Throughout that summer, Mom's symptoms presented themselves in bits and pieces, without ever revealing themselves entirely. I saw flashes and glimpses that something was wrong, but I never had enough information to fully understand what was happening. Even specialized, experienced doctors couldn't explain her symptoms or draw any logical conclusions from them.

The most frequent, prevalent symptom she experienced was fatigue. As a teenager, I struggled to understand and relate to her fatigue. I understood the idea of being tired, but I couldn't understand why she seemed to get so tired with such frequency. Was she just being lazy? Couldn't she power through? Did she really need another nap?

One particular summer day, Mom and I went to the mall to buy me new school clothes. We successfully made it to Hollister and Abercrombie, and I purchased a few shirts that I liked, but I still wanted to find a new jacket. As we walked out of Express with jeans, but still no jacket, I was mentally checking items off my list and thinking about where I still needed to go. Then I caught a glimpse of Mom and instantly froze in my tracks.

She looked at me with sadness in her eyes and exhaustion written all over her body. Her shoulders hunched forward and she couldn't seem to lift her neck straight up. She put her arm on my shoulder as I searched the aisle of the crowded mall, trying to locate the nearest bench where I could sit her down. The closest one was about fifty feet away, and I could tell she was suddenly too tired to walk that far. Instead, I helped her shuffle the two feet in front of us to the railing of the balcony. She leaned on it, looking down at the first floor of the mall, while I waited, stunned, confused, and a little agitated. I hadn't planned on this time-out. I didn't understand why it was needed, and I still had places we needed to get to.

I examined her while still gripping her shoulders, unable to let go of her for fear that she might lose her balance or fall over. She gripped tightly to the balcony railing, using all of her remaining energy to keep herself upright.

"I need to go home," she choked. I stared at her in disbelief, hoping that maybe the feeling would pass if we stood there a few moments longer.

"Seriously?" I replied. It had been an hour. *One* hour. Grandmothers could stand for longer periods of time than that.

"I'm sorry," she replied, as I felt a swell of rage form inside of me. I didn't want to leave. I wasn't even close to finished with shopping. For a moment, I just stared at her, the way disapproving teenagers do, trying desperately to convey how angry she was making me. *Seriously, Mom, you are the absolute worst.* I burned my dirtiest look into her temples, thinking that if she knew how she was making me feel, then she might reconsider her request to leave.

But she didn't reconsider. She just looked back at me, her eyes wide, sad, honest. She looked broken. It was like her eyes shot a spark of electricity at me. It hit me hard, instantly transforming my rage to sadness. Suddenly, all I felt was disappointed.

With my arm still around her shoulders, I carried her through the mall, into Macy's, in between the aisles and crowds of people, past mothers and daughters who were leisurely browsing every item on every rack without a care in the world. Finally, we made it to our car, and I drove us home to safety.

When we arrived home, Mom sang out loud to me, "Home again, home again, jiggity jig!" This was the phrase she repeated every time we pulled into the driveway. It didn't matter if we were on a week-long vacation or if we had just gone on a quick trip to the grocery store. Those words, sung in pure delight, reminded me that we were indeed officially home safe and sound. We were at Mom's favorite place in the world: home. Where everything was familiar, warm and filled with love. There was no place Mom would rather

How's Your Mom?

be than her home.

Ugh, she's such a nerd, I thought as she said it, and rolled my eyes. *Why did she have to say that every* single *time we got home?*

Dad met us at the door right away. "Hey, my girls are back! How was shopping?" he asked, a wide smile stretched across his thin lips.

"Good," I said, a little rudely. "Mom's tired."

I spared telling him the details, like how much it hurt me when I saw other moms and daughters who didn't have to leave the mall, and how confused I was by the whole episode. I pushed past Dad, who remained oblivious to my attitude.

He wrapped his arms around Mom's shoulders, the way I had done in the mall. "You're tired again?" he asked. "Do you need to take a nap?" He didn't sound annoyed like I had wanted him to. Didn't he realize we were home early? Didn't he see how obnoxious Mom was being? He acted like it was completely normal for people her age to need naps after shopping.

"Well, okay," Mom responded. "A nap would be nice. Just a quick one."

I stood there, holding my shopping bags, and watched Dad drag Mom's tired body to bed.

She stayed in bed for the entire afternoon and night.

The following day, Mom said, "I'm sorry about shopping, Shell. Did you get everything you needed?"

I didn't, but my anger from the previous day had dissipated, so I was able to contain some of my attitude. "Don't apologize. I got everything I needed," I lied. I made a mental note to go to Target by myself that night to pick up the rest of the items on my list.

"It's fine, Mom. Don't worry about it. I get it," I lied. I turned my back on her and marched away without thinking twice.

It didn't make any sense to me, and thinking about the whole thing only made me mad.

After that day, it was like she thought that if she didn't talk about her symptoms with me, then they couldn't hurt me anymore. After that episode, she began trying to hide her symptoms from me. She simply pretended like her symptoms didn't exist, like they weren't impacting my life, and did her best to carry on like everything was fine.

But it wasn't fine. Somehow *not* talking about them made everything even worse. I never had the courage to bring up anything related to her condition, so I relied on her to voluntarily tell me how she was really doing . . . but she didn't want to. She wouldn't bring it up again. Not after she saw how I responded the first time.

I was rude and scared, but it didn't mean that I didn't want to know. She talked to Dad about everything that was happening, but never to Alex or me. I would catch fragments of her conversations with Dad about her vision being wonky, or a tingly feeling she felt in her neck. But she never talked to me about anything that was happening. Was it because she didn't want to hurt me? Was she afraid of what the symptoms might mean for her future? Was she afraid because she thought I was afraid?

While she wished that she could hide her symptoms from me, I wished that she would talk to me about them.

I always thought that Mom and I were the real deal. We were *real* best friends, unlike all those other girls who liked to *pretend* their mom was their best friend. Mine really was.

For as long as I could remember, I'd always had the freedom to tell her whatever I wanted without hesitation. We never needed to hide anything from each other. She knew everything there was to know about me, even if I didn't always want her to. When I asked her how she knew so much about me, she'd reply, "Because I'm the moth-a. I know everything."

For most of my life, I thought this was a two-way street. But now, I realized I was wrong. And it wasn't fair. Why couldn't I know and understand everything about her, too?

₋₋*₋*₋*₋*

When I was little, she knew how much I hated talking out loud. We communicated a lot through writing instead. Because of our mutual love of writing, she bought us a small, soft-cover journal from the Hallmark store and told me it was for us to write back and forth. It was decorated with watercolor orange and yellow flowers on the front and back covers. When she wrote her first letter to me in 1998, when I was in second grade, the price tag was still on the back cover. It had cost twelve dollars. At the time, I thought twelve dollars was a lot of money to spend on a book with empty pages. I pondered its potential to be something special if Mom was willing to pay that much money for it. It turned out to be the most special book I would ever own.

As I progressed through elementary school, we filled the pages with our honest perceptions of our lives. At first, I wrote in it frequently, though she didn't always respond to each entry. I thought she wasn't writing because she didn't know what to write about. I'd tell her, "You can write about ANYTHING!" I'd even give her prompts, like *maybe if you have a bad day at work, you could tell me about it, and if I have a bad day at school I could tell you about it?*

Now, I couldn't help but wonder if the reason she had such a hard time writing to me was that she didn't want to talk about herself. Maybe she really just wanted to use the book as a way to get information out of me. Maybe she never intended for it to be a two-way street.

As the years went on, though, Mom did write in our book. She tried to capture all of Alex's and my huge milestones, like our bar and bat mitzvahs, graduations from high school and college, when I finished student teaching and when Alex earned his private pilot's license. Every entry ended with her telling me how much she loved us. She'd remind me that I was "the light of her life," Alex was "the beat of her heart," and Dad was "the glue that held us all together." She'd close each letter with the lyrics to our song: "I hope you dance!"

Throughout junior high and high school, a few months could pass at a time where neither of us wrote anything in our book. It wasn't intentional; we just forgot it existed sometimes. Sometimes even a few years would go by before one of us would rediscover it again, almost as if by magic. We would find it in the back of a drawer or beneath one of our beds. It would be a little dusty, and we would re-read the entire book and then feel compelled to write in it again. Every time we wrote, we would be a little more amazed at how much time had passed.

Mysteriously, she never wrote a word about the marathon she ran. Saying that she *loved* running was an understatement. She *lived* to run. So why didn't she write about her marathon? Was she too busy to document it? Was she so tied up with work, our family, and training that stopping to write it all down seemed too huge a task? Or did she not want to burden me with the details of her life? Maybe she thought being a "good mom" meant not talking about herself.

This simple, twelve-dollar, hardcover book became a symbol of my childhood. It contained all of all of the accomplishments and sorrows we both endured together: my first broken heart. My curiosity about whether or not high school love could be real. My first night at college. My heartache when my best friends turned their backs on me. When I first met the man I would come to marry. It was all there . . . I told her everything.

I told *her.*

I never once stopped to think about what she wasn't telling me.

We had both agreed that things that were hard to talk about would be easier to discuss if they were written down, rather than spoken aloud. That's why our book was so important in our relationship. It gave us the space to say whatever we needed, whenever we needed. Or, maybe, it gave *me* the space *I* needed.

Sometimes our emotions got the best of us, and we didn't always have time to pause and write things down. Instead, especially in my pre-teen years, we were forced into talking about things out loud. When I was in fifth grade, I received my first failing grade on a geography test. I had scored a sixty-four. *Sixty-four!* Never in my life had I scored a grade so low. It even had the letter "F" in bold red marker written across the top of it. (Note to teachers everywhere: don't use red ink to grade papers. Just don't. There is nothing nice about the color red on an assignment.)

Mom knew I was upset from the way I stormed into the

house, threw my backpack down and dodged her eye contact and incessant questions about how my day was. After asking "How was school?" and "Did you learn anything new today?" and getting nowhere, she knew school wasn't fine, and she knew I needed to talk, even though I wouldn't dare admit it out loud.

She called them "Danny Tanner moments," for obvious reasons if you were around in the 1990s. I was obsessed with the show *Full House* when I was growing up. At the end of every episode, Danny Tanner would walk into one of his daughters' bedrooms, explain all of the confusing parts of life to them, soft music would play, someone would cry, everyone would make up and then everything was magically all better again. Mom loved doing the exact same thing.

I didn't tell her I failed my test. I didn't have to. She didn't make me admit it out loud. It was like she already knew. Without saying a word, I turned toward my bedroom and slowly began walking away from her. With every step I took, I hoped that she would follow. I wouldn't admit that I wanted her to follow me. No teenager wants to admit how much they need their mom.

I made it all the way up the stairs and into my bedroom. When I turned around to close the door behind me, I peeked over my shoulder to see if she had followed me. She wasn't there. I buried my head in my pillow and silently wished she would follow me. Moments ticked by, but it felt like an eternity. Finally, I heard a knock on my door and a soft voice asking if I needed to have a Danny Tanner moment. I never once said, "Yes please, I'd love to have a Danny Tanner moment!" because . . . seriously, how lame would that have been?

Instead, I just looked into her eyes and hoped she would read my mind. And like any good mom could, she did. She always read my mind. She always knew when to sit down and what to say in order to make my life feel manageable again. She told me she didn't care about my test. That one test wasn't the end of the world, and my life would still go on. Or something like that. I don't remember exactly. I just know she made me feel better.

˷˷*˷*˷*

Now, as I struggled with my mother's silence about her symptoms, I understood why we called those moments "Danny Tanner moments" and not "Michelle Tanner" or "Stephanie Tanner" or "DJ Tanner" moments. They were named for the strong, all-knowing father, who initiated each meaningful conversation and always knew how to fix his daughters' problems. The daughters weren't supposed to solve the parents' problems. It was supposed to be the other way around. That's just how life was supposed to go.

I knew a lot of girls called their mom their best friend, but I could never believe that anyone could possibly be as close as Mom and I. But if it was true that we were *the real deal*, then why did she insist on hiding her symptoms from me?

CHAPTER FOUR

CHRIS

Tammy and I were high school sweethearts. I met her in the fall of 1978, the year I graduated from high school, as Tammy was entering her senior year of high school. In the spring of 1978, I took Tammy's friend, Helen, to my senior prom. Helen and I dated for a little while, but that wasn't saying much. Helen dated everybody.

The day I met Tammy, she showed up at Timmy Blackwold's house in Needham, Massachusetts, with my then ex-girlfriend, Helen. The party was like any high school house party in the seventies . . . full of teenagers smoking, drinking, and having a great time. Tammy was sitting at the kitchen table when I sat down next to her.

There was a car magazine on the table in front of us, and Tammy picked it up and began leafing through the pages, commenting on the cars featured inside. She sounded like she knew what she was talking about, and I actually believed her. How was I supposed to know she was making it all up just trying to impress me? She sounded like an expert! She totally faked me out.

Our conversation about cars turned into other easy conversations, and before we knew it, the party was winding down. At the end of the night, I asked Helen for Tammy's number, and she gave it to me. I still remember it: 769-1923. The next day, I gave her a call, which was really saying something because I never called anybody. But something in my head said, *I have got to call this girl.*

On our first date, I picked Tammy up at her split-entry house in Norwood, Massachusetts. The first thing I saw when I pulled into her driveway was her mother standing at the top of the landing looking down at me, clearly wondering what my intentions were with her daughter. I can't remember if she said anything to me, but I'll always remember the look she gave me. It was like *who are you?* I knew right away that I liked her mother. Everyone did. She didn't bother anybody. There was nothing about her not to like.

She invited me inside and asked me to sit at the kitchen table with her. Tammy's father walked into the kitchen and joined us. I introduced myself and told them a little bit about me. They must have thought I was all right because they let me take their little baby girl out to the movies that night.

We dated through the winter and spring. We used to go to the movies in Dedham, Massachusetts, a lot. We saw the original *Star Wars* together. I took her to see a movie called *The Deer Hunter*. She thought it was horrible . . . there was so much killing, blood, and guts. I thought it was beautiful. I always took her to the movie I wanted to see because I was the one driving. I played Asteroids in the arcade before the movie started. She'd stand there, patiently watching me, letting me have my fun.

In 1979, Tammy graduated from high school and began attending Bridgewater State College. I had been working as a contractor at a power plant and used to stay over in her dorm room on the weekends. It was a lot better than sleeping on the pull-out couch in her parents' basement like I had done the year before.

The following year, I was transferred to another nuclear power plant in Louisiana. Around the time of Mardi Gras, the history club at Tammy's school decided to take a trip to New Orleans. Tammy's friend asked her and a few other friends to go down with them. She said yes because she knew it would give her a chance to see me.

We had a nice week. She must have spent three days cleaning my apartment. I didn't know you were supposed to change the bed sheets. One day, we went to the Louisiana Zoo. I got a picture of a monkey giving us the finger. No. It wasn't a monkey. It was a baboon. It was a man-eating baboon. It was giving us the finger! It was beautiful.

As the week wound down, I knew I couldn't let that girl get away. She was hot, and she had no idea, which made her even hotter. So I picked up a small diamond ring at a pawn shop in Louisiana, and I asked her to marry me. I told her I knew I couldn't lose her.

She was still in college, and her mother had told her that she couldn't get married until she finished college. A true mama's girl, she wouldn't go against her mother's wishes. She turned me down, but she wanted to keep the ring. Instead of calling it an *engagement ring*, it would be a *promise ring*. I went along with it, and she wore that ring until she graduated from college.

Finally, after her graduation, she told me that she was ready to get married, and like all women, she had her dream engagement ring all pictured in her mind. She wanted a sapphire engagement ring with small diamonds on the sides. She told me that Princess Diana wore a similar ring on a much larger scale. Well, I saved up enough money to buy one for her, and one evening after dinner, in the parking lot of a restaurant, I gave it to her. She said it was exactly what she wanted. We were truly in love.

*_*_*_*_*_*_*

Before we were married, I promised her mother, Reva, that I would take care of her daughter. I didn't know exactly what the future had in store for us. But I knew, above all else, that I loved Tammy with all my heart and soul. I wanted her mother to know there was nothing in the world that would make me happier than to be her husband.

It wasn't easy to show her parents how committed I really was. Tammy was born and raised in an orthodox Jewish home. This meant that they ultimately wanted Tammy to marry a nice Jewish man. I was born and raised in an Irish Catholic family. We went to church every Sunday and said grace before each meal. When Tammy finished college and was finally ready to marry me, she asked me to convert to Judaism. She said she would have married me even if I didn't convert, but I told her I wanted to.

Trying to find a rabbi to marry us wasn't an easy task because I wasn't Jewish yet. My orthodox conversion ceremony was a week before our wedding. I had to take evening classes for a few weeks prior to the ceremony at a nearby synagogue. During the ceremony, the rabbi made me take a ritual bath to unbaptize me, and I had to have a ritual circumcision. It was a small, private service with Tammy's dad and a few others. I think I made her dad proud.

The promise to practice Judaism was one of the most important decisions I ever made in my life. But maybe even more important was the promise I made to Reva that I would take care of her daughter. I was young, dumb and in love, and I had no idea what *taking care of her* would entail, and at such a young age. But if Reva were still around today, I would make the same promise all over again.

CHAPTER FIVE
TAMMY

Since I didn't know what was causing my symptoms, I tried to tackle each complaint by seeing the doctor relevant to it.

I thought maybe the drop foot was because something was wrong with my foot. I met with a podiatrist, who told me that if I really thought it was something in my foot, he would give me a special boot to wear. He took x-rays, which, of course, revealed nothing. He told me there was nothing wrong with my foot, so I declined to wear the boot.

My primary care physician was very sympathetic toward my cause. She wanted to find a solution, and she honestly believed there was something wrong with me. "I think I have some kind of virus," I explained. "I'm just so tired. Sometimes, I lay down, put my arms across my chest, and don't even have the energy to move my arms."

"Well, let's take some blood samples," she responded. She proceeded to order every possible blood test that she could think of. Then she had me lay flat for a few minutes and then quickly rise, and immediately took my vitals. They looked perfectly fine. A few days later, most of my blood samples came back normal, too, except for one, which raised a red flag high enough to warrant sending me to a rheumatologist—a kind, middle-aged woman who encouraged me to think positively. "Blood tests often give false positives," she told me after she couldn't find anything wrong. She sent me for more blood tests and for MRIs. A few weeks later, I sat in her office as she went over everything in my records, keeping my fingers crossed that she would see something that revealed the problem. I just wanted her to figure it out. Instead, she said I was a mystery to her.

Even though she couldn't find anything wrong with me, she encouraged me to continue searching for answers. "Don't give up," she called to my back as I walked out of her office for the last time. "Keep trying to find what's wrong. Eventually, you'll come across someone who says, *Snap! I've got it!*"

In the spirit of not giving up, she referred me to a doctor in Boston. The doctor was a neurologist who was still in school. My primary care doctor had thought maybe this new, young, up-and-coming doctor would have some novel ideas.

Instead, I left that doctor's office with a diagnosis of migraines. I wanted to believe my only problem was migraines, but I didn't think it was true. It didn't make sense to me, and I didn't want to take drugs that weren't absolutely necessary. Still, I was hopeful that maybe somebody had finally found the answer. I received a prescription for amitriptyline. Although I didn't like the idea of taking drugs, I took them anyway. But I also decided to go to a doctor of osteopathic medicine, who I thought *for sure* would figure out what was wrong with me and provide me with a more natural treatment.

"I can't run anymore," I cried to him, as I explained my symptoms for what felt like the thousandth time.

"Are you under any stress at home?" he asked me.

I couldn't be sure, but it sounded like he was insinuating that my symptoms were because I was too stressed.

"Take the amitriptyline as prescribed," he recommended.

Seriously? Wasn't his job to provide *natural* solutions? Wasn't it every doctor's job to find the root cause of symptoms? He honestly thought *stress* was causing my symptoms?

"I thought you would be able to help me," I admitted shyly.

"I am helping you. You have migraines because you're stressed. You're doing this to yourself."

Stunned, I stood and walked out the door, feeling angry and disappointed that I was no closer to the truth.

A few weeks later, I visited with my primary care doctor again, and this time, she referred me to a neurologist.

Instead of seeing that doctor, however, I was seen by her assistant. She was quite thorough and asked me many questions. I must have been there for an hour. She consulted the doctor and came back twenty minutes later.

"Do you find yourself getting angry at times?" she asked.

I looked at her blankly and paused for a moment. "Of course I get angry at certain times. I'm angry right now because I'm hungry!" I snapped at her. What a ridiculous thing to ask someone!

"Well, I looked at your MRI. I noticed some white spots on your brain. I think those are what might be causing your migraines."

I still had no idea how anger would have been related to my migraines, but it didn't matter because I didn't actually have either one.

My quest continued with an appointment with a neurosurgeon. He convinced me that the tingling in my neck and arm was due to a problem with my cervical spine. He further convinced me that having a fusion in my neck would solve all my problems. It would require one night in the hospital. I readily agreed, as I was sure it would cure all that was ailing me.

The idea of having a surgical procedure to fix all that was broken delighted my entire family. We were all filled with hope and couldn't wait for me to have the surgery and be cured.

The surgery came and went, and in the weeks to follow, I had no changes in any of my symptoms. I couldn't believe it. I truly thought the doctors had found the answer. But they hadn't. Instead, I continued living day to day, trying to mask my symptoms from myself, my family, and my coworkers.

Another doctor thought something was wrong with my back. For that reason, I saw a chiropractor twice a week. After every visit, I would swear I was all better. When I ran the following day, sometimes I felt better, but other times the run would end in the same manner, with the bouncing horizon and me in a puddle of tears sitting on my doorstep wondering what was wrong with me. My chiropractor actually believed there was something wrong with me. At one point, he noticed nystagmus in my eyes. One of my eyes was moving rapidly and uncontrollably from side to side. It came and went every so often. He said something was wrong but that it was more than he could handle. He told me not to give up and to find another doctor could give me an answer.

The same thing happened when I went to an acupuncturist. She believed me when I said there was something wrong with me, but she said she felt like she was throwing darts because she had nothing to go on in placing her needles aimlessly all over my body.

My primary care doctor also sent me to an audiologist, who performed all kinds of tests on me. From reading an eye chart to having me lay flat while he poured water in my ear and telling me to recite the alphabet, his tests all seemed to try every possible thing to make the devil rise. To make "it" happen. He had me stand on the pillow and close my eyes and march in place. He put his hand on my shoulder so I wouldn't fall. I started out looking at one wall, but when I was done and opened my eyes, I had turned about forty-five degrees and was looking at another wall. I did not even know I moved. That venture ended with a basic hearing test, a diagnosis of vestibular neuritis—an inner ear infection—and a referral to see a doctor in Boston.

By that point, I was so sick of doctors that I couldn't bring myself to go.

I had been working as an optician at Nashua Eye Professionals for eight years when my symptoms first started showing. As an optician, I dealt with people's eyeglasses and eyeglass prescriptions. I translated the prescription so the patient understood it, then asked the patient how they intended to use their glasses so I could find the most appropriate glasses to fit their needs. There were several opticians on my team, and we all worked well together. I considered many of them my friends.

They all knew there was something wrong with me. They saw the way I walked, a little wobbly like I had a boozy lunch every day. They watched me hold onto the walls and counters as I moved around. They knew I was searching for a doctor to find the reason behind all of this.

Once, as I was holding onto the desk at the technician's station where technicians process paperwork and patients order contact lenses, one of the technicians eyed me cautiously as I tried to pass by. "Tammy!" she called out to me. I refrained from my crawl along the counter and looked at her.

How's Your Mom?

"I have a doctor I could recommend for you," she said. "I like him a lot. He's a little quirky, and he's a little different. Maybe he can help you. I've had various problems, and he solved what was wrong with me. Maybe he can help you, too."

I was willing to go to anyone. She made him sound very promising. Even more so, his office was in the same building where we worked. I made an appointment that very same day.

When I got to his office, I noticed how small it was. It was similar to many of the others I had been in. There was the usual stack of magazines, a row of chairs and a glass window, behind which sat the secretary. She saw me come in and slid open the glass doors so I could approach her. I told her my name and the time of my appointment, and she handed me the usual forms to fill out. I had filled out so many of those forms at the various medical offices I had already been to that I could fill them out without much thought. I returned the clipboard to the secretary, and she informed me that the doctor would be right with me. Since there was no one else in the waiting room, I knew I would be next.

The doctor came out to get me himself. Most offices have nurses escort patients into rooms, but in this case, it was just the doctor. He brought me to his office so we could have the usual pleasantries and get to know each other a little better.

He left me sitting in this office for a few moments, so I looked around the room. He had many family pictures hanging on the wall along with the usual credentials and diplomas. He had a bookcase full of books and knickknacks. I surmised from all of this that he came from Israel, and my hopes rose even more. I was certain this guy would figure out what was wrong with me. The stars were in alignment as I ticked off the reasons for my hopefulness. His office was in the same building where I worked, he was Jewish, his background was from Israel . . . enough reasons to make my spirits soar.

I noticed a huge stack of patient records on his desk, so that made me think he had a large following of patients. He returned a few moments later and sat down to begin the preliminary interview. He asked the regular questions, and I smiled as I answered my age, marital status, kids and their ages. Michelle was eighteen, Alex was twenty-one.

Then we got to business, and he asked what brought me there. I had this part all planned out in my head, and I informed him of my story and various wacky symptoms. The tingling in my neck and arm, the bouncing horizon when I ran, the foot drop, and the unbearable fatigue. I told my story and managed not to cry.

"Let's go to the exam room," he instructed. I followed him out of his office and into an adjacent room, where he handed me a gown and told me to remove my clothes. A few moments later, he came back, and the usual exam began.

"Follow my finger with my eyes."

I did as I was told.

"I'm going to test your reflexes." He banged a tiny hammer on each of my knees, but neither one responded. That wasn't a surprise, really. My reflexes had never been very responsive.

"Put your arms straight out. Hold them straight while I try to push them down," he ordered. I listened and did as he asked. Easy.

He used a needle to prick my legs with a needle. "Do you feel this?"

"Yes," I replied.

"Do you feel this?" he asked as he poked in a new spot.

"Yes," I said again.

Next, he rubbed his hands over the glands in my neck. "Don't mind my scar," I said casually. He looked at me oddly, so I continued. "I had neck surgery recently."

He didn't respond. He just gave me a funny look, like he didn't approve or didn't understand.

The neurological exam concluded with the obligatory listening to the heart and lungs. "Okay, exam over!" he snapped. "Get dressed and meet me in my office."

A few moments later, I met him in his office as he filled out a form for me to get a few more blood tests. He explained them to me, but I didn't care enough to listen. It had all been done before. Nonetheless, I wanted to believe he added a few extra labs and that he was hot on the trail of a diagnosis for me. So I took my lab order and off I went.

By this time, and by that doctor, I'd had so many blood tests I don't even know where I went to get this order filled. But when the results came back, I dutifully made an appointment for a follow-up. This time when he took me into his office, it was more familiar, so I felt completely comfortable when he entered the room. He looked over his notes to remind himself who I was and why I was there. He said a few words of introduction then he asked, "Have you ever heard of Munchausen syndrome?"

I had not.

"Well, Google it when you get home," he told me.

I said I would.

"The blood tests are completely normal. They don't show anything. I can do more tests if you want me to, but I don't see anything physically wrong," he said with a dismissive, detached tone in his voice.

"Oh," I replied, feeling completely deflated. At least he had given me a little information, but he wouldn't tell me what Munchausen syndrome was. "No, I don't want to do any more tests. Thanks anyway."

He walked me out of his office to the receptionist. There was a bowl of pistachios sitting on the ledge of the receptionist window, and as I said good-bye, I watched his large hand grab a handful. For a moment I watched him as he shelled them with his hands and tossed them casually into his mouth. Something about it struck me as odd, and a complete turn-off. I made an appointment for a third visit, though I knew I wouldn't keep it. He had nothing more to offer me.

When I arrived home that night, as promised, I looked on my computer to see what Munchausen syndrome was. As I read the results, I couldn't believe my eyes. *This must be a dream.* I immediately burst into tears.

I learned that Munchausen syndrome afflicts people who seek out different doctors for non-existent conditions that they have constructed in their minds. This doctor had diagnosed me with a mental illness. He had told me it was all in my mind.

I'm not saying mental illnesses aren't very real, serious conditions. They are. But it's not what had. I was *not* doing this to myself.

My crying must have been loud because my daughter heard me all the way from the kitchen. "Mom?" She leaned on the doorframe and poked her head into my bedroom. "What's wrong?"

I motioned for her to come in, then cried to her uncontrollably as I explained the Munchausen syndrome diagnosis. I watched her reaction, trying to figure out if she believed I was making it all up, too.

"It's not all in my mind. You believe me, don't you?" I asked her feebly. What if she didn't? What if she thought the doctor was right? What would I do if my own daughter didn't even believe in me?

"Mom, you're not making this up," she stated, her hazel eyes staring directly into mine. She sat next to me as a few silent moments ticked by.

"Just keep seeing doctors," she told me. "Someone will figure it out."

~~*~*~*~*

About a year later, in 2009, I met that pistachio-eating doctor in the elevator of our shared building. By that point, I had progressed to using a cane. As I hobbled into the elevator, I felt him shrink backwards into the wall of the elevator. He remembered me; I knew he did. He looked me up and down, and I scowled back at him.

Munchausen syndrome. I *wished* that was all I had.

He couldn't look me in the eye. Mercifully, the elevator ride was short, but he couldn't get out fast enough. As soon as the elevator pinged on the ground floor, he rushed through the doors and never once looked back at me—the woman who was just making it all up.

CHAPTER SIX

CHRIS

We had a pretty simple life. Things were good. Easy. We didn't need much. We didn't bother anybody.

Then, suddenly, around 2007, things weren't fine anymore. We knew something was wrong, but for months, nobody was able to figure it out.

I was pissed. The so-called "professionals" kept giving Tammy MRIs at a thousand dollars a whack. They kept telling us that they knew what the issue was. They said they could fix it if we let them operate on her. They unnecessarily put her through a serious operation, and she was scheduled for another. That's why they called it "practicing" medicine—because they really didn't know what they were doing.

I have to give it to them . . . they did try. But they kept wanting to operate on her instead of trying to find out what the root cause was. And we trusted them. We kept thinking she would be fine if we let the doctors operate on her.

But one day, on her way to work, Tammy rear-ended someone with her Mazda. That's when I started freaking out.

She *totaled* that car. The guy in front of her stopped short, and her front bumper slammed right into his. She told me later that she couldn't stop. She told me her foot was numb, and that's why she couldn't feel the brake. That's why she rear-ended the guy. That's why she almost got herself killed.

She got his information, but I think he was an illegal alien because he didn't really want to stick around. It was a good thing for us that he didn't do anything because he could have sued the pants off of her for rear-ending him.

Anyway, that was when it started. We still didn't have any answers, but for someone to suddenly not be able to control their leg while they were driving a vehicle told me that something was wrong. I'd had enough of those doctors throwing fucking darts, hoping one would hit the bullseye. I could have done that. Once she totaled that car, I knew this was something we had to get figured out.

I marched her into her primary care doctor's office and saw the doctor who was on call. I told the doctor that if he didn't find out what was wrong with my wife, then I was going to start shooting people, starting with him.

(No, I wouldn't have actually shot the guy. Relax. You can't carry a gun in a hospital.)

He went out of his mind. "You can't say that to me!" he yelled. Tammy started freaking out, instructing me to calm down.

"Listen," I said, staring into his eyes, standing an inch away from his face, towering over him. "There's something wrong with her, and you fucking assholes aren't figuring it out."

"I'll examine her again," he told us reluctantly.

"Damn right, you will," I scoffed as we followed him into an examination room.

After a thorough examination, he agreed to send a referral to another doctor who worked in a small gray building on the corner of Main Street in our hometown.

We immediately drove over.

We waited eagerly in the waiting room. A couple of minutes later, the doctor walked in. He was wearing leather sandals and a Hawaiian-print, button-down shirt. His hair was tied in a ponytail that reached past his waist.

Listen, I didn't like Hawkeye on *M*A*S*H*. The minute this guy came walking out, I thought *this isn't going to fucking go well.*

"Take it easy," Tammy instructed, reading my mind.

He led us toward the examination room but stopped us in the hallway to watch Tammy walk with her cane. He asked her to put her cane down and walk down the hallway, using the railings mounted to the walls on each side if necessary.

She took a few steps, and he said, "I think you have MS." Just like that.

He instructed us to visit another doctor at a hospital in Lebanon, New Hampshire, to confirm the diagnosis. I didn't know

How's Your Mom?

much about MS, but I knew it could be bad. I knew that there was no cure. I knew she would probably never get better.

I had a lot of questions, and I was wicked pissed off and scared, even though I didn't dare admit it out loud.

We walked out of that building, got into the car, and immediately headed for Lebanon. By the time we reached the interstate in my Ford Crown Victoria, we were both crying. My tears only fueled the car, and the more anger and pain rose inside of me, the faster I drove.

"Slow down!" Tammy yelled at me, a panicked, urgent constriction in her voice.

I couldn't slow down. Instead of letting up on the gas, I put the fucking throttle right to the floor.

When my speedometer read 120 miles per hour, I finally thought, *I better slow down.*

When we arrived at the hospital thirty-five minutes later, we found out for the very first time just how bad MS really was, how badly it could hurt you.

PART TWO
MAKING AN OFFER
NOVEMBER 2009–AUGUST 2015

CHAPTER SEVEN

CHRIS

My mind raced as the doctor spoke to us in his office. So many thoughts spun around in my head. Some of them terrified me, others gave me hope.

I wanted to know just how bad multiple sclerosis really was. Did it mean she was going to die?

I also couldn't help but feel relieved and grateful for *finally* having a diagnosis.

Was it treatable? Would she get better? Stay the same? Get worse?

Questions continued racing through my mind like a race car speeding around a track. They just whirled around and around, until something finally crashed, and one of the cars caught fire.

" . . . you'll have about six months to a year . . ." I heard the doctor say.

WHAT? My head jerked up, and my eyes felt like they popped out of their sockets. I didn't speak. I couldn't speak if I wanted to. Had I really heard him say that?

" . . . until you'll be in a wheelchair," he finished.

Oh, a wheelchair.

Wait, *a wheelchair*?! *Six months? This guy has to be out of his mind.*

Let me make this clear: I am not a crier. I don't cry. I hunt, fish, work on classic cars, and do all kinds of masculine things. Crying isn't one of them.

Before that moment, I hadn't cried since my mom's funeral, which had been seven years before. But there I was, standing in a doctor's office, crying like a baby. Even I could barely believe it.

The doctor kept talking, but I couldn't hear him. I just said "yeah" every now and then and kept nodding my head.

After what felt like hours, the doctor finally rose to his feet, and we immediately did the same. I shook his hand, and he hand-ed me a small plastic bag, which appeared to be full of papers and stuff. He had probably just explained what was inside; I hadn't been listening.

Fortunately, Tammy was paying very close attention. Once we were in the car, she explained to me that the bag of crap wasn't crap at all. It was actually filled with important reading material, pamphlets about MS, and information about the drug that he recommended she start on. The drug was called Betaseron, and it was to be taken as an injection once per day. A nurse would be in touch with us soon to set up an appointment to teach us how to use the medicine.

In both of our minds, we thought the diagnosis was the end. It turned out, it was only the beginning.

How's Your Mom?

CHAPTER EIGHT
MICHELLE

I was home when my parents returned from the hospital in Lebanon. They casually dropped a little goody bag on the counter in the kitchen. Then they walked away, heading for their bedroom so Mom could rest.

I crept into the kitchen and peeked curiously into the bag. I picked it up and pulled out a brochure for a drug called Betaseron. This gave me a surge of hope; at the very least, she was already on a treatment plan for whatever she had. Surely that was a good sign. Then I learned that Betaseron was a drug for treating multiple sclerosis. *Multiple sclerosis.* I had never heard of it. I deduced that must be what the doctors decided she had.

I continued digging through the bag and found another pamphlet entitled "All About Multiple Sclerosis." I pulled it out, unfolded the pages, and lay it flat on the counter in front of me. I took a few deep breaths, knowing this brochure was about to outline all the answers I needed but didn't really want to know. I blinked hard, then began to read.

The first thing that caught my eye was a graphic image of a timeline. It was idiot-proof and perfectly designed. Someone must have spent a lot of time designing it. Tears immediately began welling up in my eyes, and I wondered if the person who created it knew the effect it would have on those who read it.

Confused and horrified by the image in front of me, I forced myself to study it, to really understand it. I needed to know what was wrong with Mom. According to the graphic, within a few years from the date of diagnosis, patients with MS usually needed a cane to walk. But Mom had just been diagnosed, and she was already using a cane. What was next?

I forced myself to move my eyes down the timeline to five years from the diagnosis. That would be the year 2014. At this point, the timeline suggested that she'd probably need a walker. When I reached the end of the timeline, ten years from diagnosis (the year 2019 for us), an image of a wheelchair glared back at me. That was it. That was where the timeline ended. It didn't, as I feared, end at death. It just ended at the wheelchair. What would my mom look like with a wheelchair? Our front porch had stairs; how would a wheelchair even work in our house? Would she be able to keep working? I had so many questions.

I blinked back the tears that were clawing their way down my face, folded the pamphlet back up and shoved it inside the bag. I made it look like I hadn't touched anything. I didn't want my parents to know what I had learned. I honestly wished I hadn't even looked. I wanted to turn back time and take the past two minutes of my life back.

But it was too late. I couldn't reverse time. I could only continue venturing into the cloudy mist that was my family's future. I could have walked into my parents' bedroom and asked them out loud. I could have talked to my parents about all of the fears and anxiety that was rising up inside of me. But I didn't want to acknowledge it. I didn't want to be anywhere near my parents.

Instead, I ran to my room, taking the steps two at a time to get there faster. I slammed my bedroom door shut and remained still as a statue for as long as I possibly could.

I couldn't think. Couldn't move. Couldn't believe any of it was real.

Maybe, if I stayed in my bedroom forever, time would freeze, and she would never get worse.

Later, it occurred to me that my parents hadn't even had the guts to tell me the name of her diagnosis out loud. Why else would they have left the goody bag on the counter for me to find? They must have *wanted* me to figure it out that way. Honestly, I didn't blame them. Even Danny Tanner wouldn't have been able to handle a conversation like that. It was probably better for me to find out through the goody bag.

The act of retreating into my bedroom became something of a habit for me. Denial and hope conflicted inside my head daily, fighting with each other constantly to come to the top of my mind. On some days, denial would win, and I successfully denied that she

How's Your Mom?

was really sick. On other days, my hopelessness got the best of me, and it was all I could do to convince myself that she was going to be fine; she wouldn't actually get worse.

For a while, Dad, Alex, and I all really believed she wouldn't let MS win. And Mom thought she would beat it, too.

CHAPTER NINE
MICHELLE

The cause of MS still remains a mystery. Sure, pharmacy companies have come out with drugs to try to treat the symptoms, but no one has been able to figure out *why* those symptoms occur in the first place. The disease, or *villain* as I sometimes called it, seems to creep into your life out of absolutely nowhere. *Something* makes the immune system attack the brain and spinal cord. This causes damage to the myelin, which is what provides insulation for the nerve fibers in the body. As a result of the damaged myelin, the communication signals become interrupted and cause symptoms like those Mom experienced, in addition to others like memory problems, blindness or paralysis.

I couldn't help but think of MS as simply an unpredictable, greedy bitch that wants to steal your life.

Everyone's experience with MS is completely different. Some patients have good days where they feel completely normal, and other days where their symptoms flare up so badly that their lives have to come to a complete halt. Other patients' symptoms are more consistent and don't change from day to day. Specifically, patients with Progressive MS who are already in a wheelchair seem to be able to expect a bit more consistency with their symptoms, but they can still suffer from "attacks" where their symptoms worsen temporarily, too.

Even though every individual disease is completely different, if there was one thing I learned, it was that once the villain attacked you, there was no escaping it.

At least, there won't be a way to escape it *successfully* until someone finds a damn cure.

How's Your Mom?

CHAPTER TEN
TAMMY

"Wow, you look really great," I said to my friend, Anne, who walked into Nashua Eye Professionals one day. She had just been diagnosed with Relapsing-remitting MS, only a few months after I had. It wasn't like me to make that type of comment to someone I only considered an acquaintance, but she looked so good that I couldn't help myself. "What are you doing to make yourself look so fit?"

"I do yoga every day and play tennis whenever I can," she replied casually. Her blonde hair looked like it had fresh highlights, and it sparkled against her tanned skin. I couldn't fathom how she could play tennis out in the sun on a hot day, knowing if I ever tried to do that, I would melt into a pile of sobbing nerves. How was it possible that we had the same disease?

The people with Relapsing-remitting MS fell victim to random flare-ups and attacks. I heard stories about people who would lose their vision for hours or days at a time, only to have it, and all other elements of normalcy, return to them as if nothing happened. When these attacks struck, they became completely unable to live their daily lives. But the attacks always subsided. They were always able to walk again.

My disease was different. I had a cane and Progressive Relapsing Multiple Sclerosis, the rarest form, which doctors knew the least about. Although I had some days where my symptoms were worse than others, my life never fully went back to normal. It was like I was constantly taking two steps backwards but only one step forward, never fully regaining what I'd lost.

After a while, I started calling Relapsing-remitting MS the *good* kind. It was the kind of MS you saw in the TV commercials . . . the kind the MS Society even used to promote strength and courage in all MS patients. Those commercials were brutal to watch. It's almost like a form of brainwashing. While you're watching, you're forced to think, *Look at them! They're still walking and fighting it!*

That means I can, too!

"You should do yoga with me sometime!" Anne cheered at me, a positive glimmer in her eyes that I couldn't look away from. "You know, I'm working toward obtaining my yoga certification," she continued before I could respond. "I need to accumulate one hundred hours of teaching. Maybe I could come over to your house, help you do yoga, and earn some hours?"

I thought about saying no, but, how could I? She looked so good that I couldn't help but wonder if yoga was really all I needed to feel better myself.

Anne came to my house four times over the course of a month to do chair yoga with me. She swore up and down that if I did this yoga, the MS wouldn't progress. I scoffed at that thought because not only had I done yoga before my MS diagnosis, I had also done Pilates, power yoga, boot camp workouts, and of course, running five miles a day.

"Do you really think it will help me?" I asked.

"It works for me, and we both have MS!" she responded.

I was glad she believed that yoga had the power to help her so exponentially, but after a few weeks of doing yoga with her, I realized it didn't hold the same power for me. During those little yoga sessions, I thanked her and oozed happiness, wishing that the yoga would be the end-all to my MS. I enjoyed the camaraderie more than anything. When a month had gone by, I was certain it didn't hold the magic answer for me.

Anne did go on to become a certified yoga instructor. Of course, she had a soft spot for the people with MS who would do yoga with her. She continued with her specialty yoga for MS, and she was proof that it certainly did work for some types of MS. Just not for the kind I had.

I continued to seek treatment for my variety of ailments in my early attempt to fight the progression. My neurologist gave me a referral to get physical therapy. I was in such good shape at that time that the physical therapy was a joke to me. Nonetheless, I went through the motions with a good attitude, saying all along that it was a huge help.

How's Your Mom?

The sessions took place at a hospital in my hometown so I could make convenient appointments before work. One physical therapist, in a valiant attempt to figure out what caused my symptoms, had me lay on the table and flop my head back and forth from side to side. She wanted to "make it happen." That's what I called those moments when the MS would rear its ugly head and do its thing: making "it" happen. The horizon would float. There would be tingling in my arm. Later on, my legs would give way, and I would end up on the floor.

We used all kinds of fancy machinery to try to make "it" happen. Unfortunately, it didn't matter when I called upon "it" to strike or asked "it" to go away. "It" came and went as it damn well pleased.

Physical therapy was covered by my insurance with one condition: I had to report that it was having an impact on my well-being. But if I were being honest, it did not have any impact for me. My physical therapist was unable to get me to the point of showing that it was improving my function. "There's nothing else we can do for you. We need to end the treatment," she told me one day, on what became my last day of physical therapy.

Insurance covered sixteen sessions with the physical therapist with the intention that you would continue to do the exercises on your own at home. It all seemed so futile to me. The progression would happen as if it had a will of its own. It seemed like it truly did not matter what I did to try to fight it. MS would probably always beat me.

*_*_*_*_*_*

The most frustrating unsolicited advice I ever received came while I was in the grocery store.

I knew that people meant well. Most of the time, people were just trying to help. But these people were neither doctors nor medical professionals, and they often knew very little about the subject matter they professed to know everything about. They had no data or factual information to back up anything they asserted to be true, they just *maybe* heard it sometime, somewhere, from someone, and thought it would be helpful to pass it on to me.

I was out grocery shopping on my own. I was patiently debating between buying two different brands of spaghetti sauce, one of which was on sale but had more sugar than its more expensive alternative. It was a tricky decision for me to make as a woman who worked very hard for every cent I earned but cared very much about everything my family and I ate.

Out of nowhere, an old acquaintance appeared at my side. She didn't know me very well, but I had a tendency to talk to everyone as though we were great friends. I tended not to hold back in conversations. I told her about my symptoms, and the many doctors I had been going to see, and the absolute lack of clarity surrounding it all.

As if it were obvious, she simply looked at me and told me, "It's the way you eat."

What the fuck? I seriously could not believe that she had just said that to me. She proceeded to tell me about her diet of only fruits and vegetables and encouraged me to reconsider the foods I put into my body. She examined my shopping cart suspiciously as I hung my head in disbelief.

Did she really think I was eating poorly? Did she think I feasted solely on sugar and processed foods? Had I not just been spending far too long trying to decide which jar of spaghetti sauce to buy because one jar had ten grams less sugar per serving?

I had also been told, in various conversations, that my MS was because of the plastic Tupperware containers where I stored my foods. I had been told it was due to the chemicals added to the fat-free versions of food I ate, like fat-free Cheez-its and fat-free Oreos. Those were the culprit.

Others told me it was due to chemicals like aspartame found in diet sodas (which I never drank) and high fructose corn syrup, which can be found in just about everything.

People loved to tell me what the problem was, as if they were the experts. The truth was that they had no more clue about what caused MS than those who were heavily involved in researching and studying it. Still, that didn't stop people from pushing their opinions onto me.

I tried to believe their opinions were rooted in the spirit of trying to help me, but it grew infuriating to listen to. Their opinions implied that my MS was something I had control over, and if only I changed certain elements of my lifestyle, I would be cured. Did they seriously think this was something I was doing to myself? What else did they think of me?

CHAPTER ELEVEN

TAMMY

A few months after my diagnosis, I was at work. It was almost two o'clock in the afternoon on a freezing cold winter day, the time when my body usually started to give up on me. Every day, around that time, it was as if my nerves simply decided to check themselves out, leaving me wanting to collapse. It was much worse than the typical mid-afternoon drowsiness I had experienced in my pre-MS days, but a completely different kind of physical, mental, and emotional exhaustion. Sometimes, it was all I could do to continue standing and not melt into a puddle of tears.

I glanced toward the clipboard containing the names of patients who were waiting to be seen by the next available optician, which lay on the opposite side of the waiting area. I walked to the clipboard, relying heavily on my cane to help me get there. I didn't mind bringing my cane to work, and it had taken only a few days to adjust to using it. It truly was a luxury to have; it made my life so much easier. I wanted to keep working, and I thought that if I focused on remaining strong, even if that meant relying on a cane, then I could fight whatever evil plans MS had for me. Who would I be without my career? How could I ever be so disabled that I couldn't work anymore? I forced the thought out of my mind, sure that I could and would never get that bad.

I picked up the clipboard and read the next name on the list in my head before saying it out loud. Just as I opened my mouth to call the name, a siren blared from the fire alarms along the walls. The lights flashed brightly, and a calm voice said, "*Attention! A fire has been detected in the building. Proceed to the nearest exit immediately.*"

I immediately glanced at my coworkers, who seemed just as surprised as I was by the interruption, although it wasn't the first time a fire alarm had gone off in our building. Construction was constantly being done in the building, and we had been told that the fire alarm might go off occasionally. We were required by law to vacate the building anytime it did. My team of opticians and I were usually glad for the little break it provided because it meant we could step outside for at least a few moments. I supposed it was bad for business and for the people who were having an eye exam, but for us, it was usually a nice little break.

Today, as the alarm sounded, a jolt of panic shot through me. As everyone else leapt to their feet and began making fast, sturdy strides toward the exit, I realized I could not move as quickly as everyone else. Others began lining up behind me, and sensing how slowly I was moving with my cane, they politely stepped around me. It wasn't rude; it was simply survival.

However, my coworker friends wouldn't leave me in the dust. Destinee, my sweet, young friend, instantly appeared at my side. "Keep walking. I'm going to grab your jacket from the break room," she told me. *Oh, sheesh. I hadn't even thought about getting my jacket.* For a normal person to get there, it shouldn't take more than ten seconds. I would have never been able to make it to the break room, which was located on the opposite side of the waiting room.

As Destinee ran to fetch our jackets, I continued hobbling toward the exit, clutching my cane fiercely so as not to fall and make everything much worse.

Another coworker, Julie, looped my free arm through hers and provided me with the extra support I needed to make it to the exit. Together, we walked to safety, and Destinee met us outside with our jackets.

As the cool air hit my face, I realized for the first time that my disability had the power to put others in jeopardy of their own safety. Had this been a real emergency, both Destinee and Julie were ready to risk their own lives to help me stay safe and get out of the building. It was the first time I realized how dependent I was becoming on others around me. And it didn't sit well with me.

What if something terrible really did happen while I was at work? Luckily, this hadn't been a real fire. But what if there really was a fire and I fell down, and someone else had to run inside to save me? What if I inadvertently put others in danger?

A few weeks later, I gave my notice that I would be leaving work on Family Medical Leave of Absence (FMLA). According to the terms of my benefits package, I was provided with four weeks' of FMLA, where my job would be considered secure while I figured out what the future held for my physical abilities. My insurance coverage would remain intact through the Consolidated Omnibus Budget Reconciliation Act (COBRA) for twelve months.

I told myself, and my family, that I needed time to process all changes that were happening in my body and determine how I would continue working with them without relying on the help of others. I would figure it out—I was sure of it. I told everyone would be back at work in just a few weeks.

But at the same time, I was growing angry at the world. I was getting incredibly sick of other people. I was sick of pretending to care. As much as I didn't want to be *forced* to stop working, in a way, I did *want* to stop working. Although, I recognized that if I stopped, it might be terrible for me. I recognized the fact that leaving work might not be temporary. It might turn into another milestone on my MS journey that I would have to look back on. So, of course, I wanted to prolong it as long as possible. But the truth was that I was so sick of people. I wanted to be left alone.

Well . . . not totally alone. I wanted my family to visit me. I liked when my kids sat with me. They picked really good movies.

When my kids visited with me, I still felt like their mother. I would sit in my chair like a perfectly normal person, holding my tea and completely forgetting the fact that my left hand was numb. Michelle would talk to me about her friends and school, and Alex would tell me about his job or the next trip he was taking with his cross-my-fingers-future-daughter-in-law, Christine. They were great kids. Chris and I always asked ourselves how we got so lucky.

Alex was my IT guy. He kept all my electronic thingys working. He was smart, patient, and didn't try to be anyone but himself. But boy, was he stubborn. Once, when he was around two years old, he was eating Cheerios in his high chair. Actually, he wasn't eating them. He was dropping them, one by one, onto the floor. With each purposeful drop, he'd look at me, like *what are you gonna do about it, Mom?*

I remembered it all so clearly. At first, I didn't say anything. I knew he was just testing me to see how much he could get away with. After the fifth Cheerio hit the floor, his smile grew so wide I couldn't take it anymore. "ALEXANDER PAUL, YOU STOP THROWING THOSE CHEERIOS RIGHT NOW!" I looked him in the eye, his lips suddenly forming a straight line. His smile faded.

Ha, I thought. *It worked.*

But one second later, his little hand was reaching for the pile of Cheerios again. This time, he picked up an entire fistful of them, then moved his hand over the edge of his chair, and slowly opened up his fist, letting all of the Cheerios fall onto the floor. His eyes never left mine. His crooked, wide smile returned. And I almost smiled with him—he was just so cute.

It was then that I learned to never try to tell Alex what to do. Telling him what to do would only make him want to do the opposite. I could motivate and encourage and try to persuade him to follow the path I thought was best, but I would never again tell my Alex what to do.

Michelle was quite different from her brother. Maybe it was simply because she was a girl, and a very unique one at that. Ever since she was little, she was nothing like the other girls, although she always wanted to be. I did not know why, but every time she became part of a group of girls, she became the odd man out. Somehow, I was sure it was my fault. I wanted her to be independent, and also compassionate and humble. Yet she always wanted to hang with the gang. The popular girls. I guess she just never really fit in with them. The qualities I was cultivating are a contradiction to those sorts of "friendships."

So, of course, it was my fault that she went through a lot of shit with friendships. She had trouble fitting in with kids in elementary school and was bullied online in middle school, and in college, her entire group of best friends and roommates suddenly turned on her. I would never understand why.

But you know what? I decided to hang tough and stay the

course. I would continue with this philosophy, encouraging her to be independent and strong, instead of trying to fit in with the crowd. I knew that she would be strong, and she would be kind. Someday she would do great things. Maybe not for the whole world, but at least for Michelle world.

Yes, I was still me. I may have to take a break from one of the most important things that defined me—my career— but I was *still me*. I was not MS. I was still *the Mom*.

CHAPTER TWELVE

MICHELLE

Mom didn't stop working all at once, but rather, she started by taking a Family Medical Leave of Absence (FMLA) . . . and she just never went back. From my perspective, it looked like she physically couldn't do it anymore. Between waking up early in the morning, preparing and packing a lunch each day, walking around all day at work, and the commute to and from, it had all become all too much for her to handle.

"Have I told you about the Spoonie theory?" she asked me on one of her first days on FMLA.

"The *what*? No," I replied shortly.

"The MS bloggers call themselves 'Spoonies.'" She paused, waiting for me to show a sign of interest. Instead, I just stared blankly back.

"Well, every day, it's like I'm given a set number of spoons. Everything I do requires me to spend my spoons. Even simple things like standing up, brushing my teeth, or walking across the room cost me a number of spoons."

"Um, okay?" I responded, too baffled by her stupid analogy to respond respectfully. What the hell was she trying to tell me?

"Once I use them all, my energy is gone," she said.

Oh. She was trying to tell me why she got so tired, I realized.

"The only way I can recharge my spoon supply is to sleep," she said.

"Right . . . okay." I turned my back on her, wanting to be finished with the conversation. She was given spoons? And when they were gone, she ran out of energy? How was this any different from the rest of us? EVERYONE GOT TIRED! The difference was, we didn't have to take naps all the time!

"I don't have enough spoons to make it through the day at work anymore," she sighed. I felt sorry for her, but I didn't know what I could do to help her or make anything better.

I realized that "career" would now be added to the List of Things—the imaginary list where we inventoried all the things MS had stolen from her. Already on the list were *running, cooking, cleaning* and *socializing regularly with friends*. I worried that *walking* would also soon appear on the List of Things.

It didn't take a genius to see that her cane wasn't enough help to her anymore. But before she transitioned completely from Candy Cane (our pet name for her cane) to a walker, which Dad purchased out of pocket and we referred to as "Little Buggy," she improvised an intermediate solution: the Tea Cart. We called it the Tea Cart because it was the place where Mom put her tea mug and biscotti as she walked, or rather dragged herself uneasily, from the kitchen to the living room each night.

By the time the Tea Cart came into our lives in 2010, I was a sophomore in college. I had just started dating Tyler, a guy I'd met at school, who was two years older than I was. I had met him at a college party the previous fall, and we began dating that spring. He met every criterion on the checklist I had written when I was twelve years old, titled "My Perfect Man." (I got the idea for the list from a book in the series called *Mates, Dates* by Cathy Hopkins that my friend, Hannah, let me borrow in sixth grade. And I ended up using the material from my list in my wedding vows, so don't make fun of me.)

Tyler was taller than me, strong but not anywhere near obsessed with fitness or his own good looks, loved his family, had a good sense of style and knew how to make me laugh. Oh, and he had clean fingernails. That was a super important trait to me. He was kindhearted and always patient with me, and he was a great listener. In many ways, he seemed too good to be true. After only a month, Tyler and I told each other we loved each other. (Okay . . . the whole story goes like this: it was about four a.m. and he was drunk when he first said it, and I didn't say it back, but I was really happy. For the entire week afterwards, I was terrified that if I brought it up, he would tell me he didn't mean it, didn't remember it, or it was a mistake. So, the following Saturday night, I got drunk and told him I loved him. Fortunately, he said it back and then asked if I remembered him saying it. *Did I remember?! Was he joking?* He explained that he couldn't remember how I had reacted, so he was too afraid to say it again just in case it scared me.) *Alcohol. Honestly.*

The important thing was that we meant it. I swear.

Anyway, Tyler was the real deal. *We* were the real deal. And I couldn't wait for my parents to meet him.

On the weekend of my birthday, April 18, he drove to my parents' house with me. We ate cake, and my parents gave me a guitar for a birthday present because I was certain that I could learn to play and be just like Taylor Swift.

I appreciated that Mom didn't try to be anyone she wasn't that weekend. She wanted Tyler to know right away what she was really like. She didn't want him to get any false impressions about her. She asked Tyler to help push her Tea Cart around the house for her while she sat in her chair, conserving her spoons. He happily obliged, not paying any attention to the fact that his girlfriend's mom was far from perfect. Actually, he seemed genuinely happy to help her. She laughed at all his jokes, and she seemed really impressed with him. The idea that my parents might really like him filled me with a warm glow. Then Dad took him downstairs to see his gun collection and warned him that he had buried my first boyfriend under the shed.

When I looked back on 2010, I realized it was a great year. We just had no idea how good we had it. The Tea Cart was a huge help for allowing Mom to get around the house. It was a form of a "walker" without her having to actually admit it. It made her feel independent. But eventually, its thin, white, metal frame and four small shelves on wheels weren't exactly safe to use as she had been doing. It surely wasn't meant to support a one-hundred-pound person leaning on it so frequently. Plus, unlike real walkers, it didn't have a place where she could sit if she needed to take a break. One day, after I had returned home for the summer, Dad just showed up at home with Little Buggy. The Tea Cart joined Candy Cane in the closet, never to be needed again, but never forgotten, either.

Eventually, her big, cozy chair in the living room became

worn-in, and within a couple months, it became the place where she spent the majority of her time. The disease spread across her whole body. She lost all feeling in her left leg and slowly began to lose feeling in her right. Just as I suspected, *walking* was added to the List of Things by the time I started my junior year of college.

Although the List of Things seemed to grow almost daily, she remained focused on the things she could still do. She *loved* the iPad that Alex purchased for her, and her days became filled with hours of Candy Crush, Words with Friends, and reading MS blogs. This was her new life—she had to learn to love it.

In 2011, about a year after Little Buggy came into our lives, it, too, was replaced. We called her wheelchair Jazzy Blue, for its brand name and the bright blue color of the base. It was like the Incredible Hulk as far as electric wheelchairs went, and it gave Mom the freedom to move around the house again. Jazzy Blue was accompanied by a smaller, manual wheelchair, which we used if we had to take her out of the house.

As the years went on, we referred to the Tea Cart as a milestone in our journey; we all marveled at how healthy Mom was when she first met Tyler. At the time, we thought the Tea Cart would be as bad as things would ever be. We thought that if she continued trying new medicines, then she wouldn't get worse. Things would only go up from there. We had no way of knowing what was really in store for us.

Even after years passed by, it all remained a mystery to me. Maybe none of it seemed real because it all happened so quickly in the grand scheme of things, and because I was away at college for most of it. The MS brochure said we would have ten years until something like Jazzy Blue would appear in our lives. Instead, we got three.

Sometimes I'd catch myself looking at Mom but not really seeing her. It was like all I could see was an empty shell of where Mom used to be. I wanted the imposter who had taken over Mom's body to go away. More than anything in the world, I just wanted Mom back. She was sitting right in front of me! But it wasn't her anymore.

How's Your Mom?

In the spirit of trying to be just like Taylor Swift, I wrote a song about all the confusing thoughts rolling around in my head. The chorus said:

When they ask, how's your mom?
I tell them I don't know,
Feels like she disappeared a couple years ago
Might look, to you, like she's sitting there
In that same worn-out chair
But that helpless person looking back at me
Is not the Mom that I used to see.
The song ended with:
They say how's your mom?
Feels like she's gone.

If you didn't know she had MS, and you just saw her sitting down in her chair, you would have no clue that she was sick. People call it an "invisible disease," because you truly would have no idea it was there if you didn't know. When most people see someone with an invisible disease, we assume they are completely healthy.

So, I did what most people did when they saw her. I made up my mind that she wasn't really sick, and I told myself that she was actually just fine. She was being dramatic.

Pretending that she was *fine* and *faking it* made it easy for me to grow angry at her. I hated that she would rather sleep than try to go to the mall with me. I was hurt when she didn't want to bake cookies with me. I thought it meant she didn't want to spend time with me. I'd get frustrated when the house looked messy and wondered why she wasn't cleaning as often she used to. When I found expired food in the refrigerator, I'd make a point to tell her that it *should have been thrown away* and tried my best to make her feel bad for forgetting to do so. I had transformed into a bitch who hated her mom . . . a girl I never thought I would be.

Eventually, everything about our new life with the villain in it made me upset. It all came down to the fact that *I* was the daughter; *she* was the mother. *She* was supposed to taking care of *me*. Not the other way around.

CHAPTER THIRTEEN

TAMMY

On my first day staying home on FMLA in February 2011, I promised to abide by one rule: Wake up at seven every morning and take a shower first thing. After that, I hoped to do some kind of activity. Maybe some housework, maybe some paperwork. Something to take care of business.

On that first morning, after waking up at seven and taking a shower, I made my way to the kitchen. Chris was there. I got some letters ready to mail and found a birthday card for my niece in my box of cards. Feeling very productive already, I decided to clean out my closet.

Chris had so many clothes and so many duplicates because instead of organizing his shit, he just bought more. I used to do the organizing for him back in the day, but it had totally gotten out of control in the past few years. *Well,* I thought, *he's going to rue the day that Queen Tammy comes back to take charge of the castle!*

I worked for about two hours until I went to spaghetti. I'd made a good dent in the closet. It was a good start.

I took a break. I walked back to the kitchen, made myself some tea, and sliced an apple. Spooned peanut butter onto my apple and started seeing double. I was unable to continue standing. I wondered how I ever made it through a day at work, then remembered that I hadn't—I would be a pile of nerves and tears by mid-afternoon. I felt a wave of gratitude for my home, as I sat so comfortably there now.

I thought about what might happen in the future, but realized I had no idea. The only thing I knew was that time would pass quickly.

On the second day of FMLA, I dragged myself out of bed at seven-fifteen. I made my way into the kitchen, expecting to feel as good as I'd felt the day before. I cleaned up the counters a little bit, but then my body went to spaghetti again. I sat at the snack bar, drinking my coffee, being careful not to guzzle, since the day before I had drunk it slowly, and I thought maybe that was the magic elixir to giving my body strength.

All of a sudden, I felt dizzy, hot, and had pain at the top of my head. *Why?*

I could not walk. I dragged my dead legs into the living room and sat in my chair. Cried a little. I felt the urge to poop, and that's the only reason I got up. I did not make it to the bathroom in time.

I dragged my body into the shower and proceeded to drop the conditioner and the shower gel before getting myself somewhat clean and finally dragging myself out again. I sat on the toilet to do my hair and managed to get dressed. All the while, I wondered *how the hell I ever made it to work.*

And then, just like that, I could walk! A switch magically got turned on, and I was walking again. Why?!

*_*_*_*_*_*

The whole first month on FMLA was difficult, sort of like I was in a tunnel. . . . just kind of drifting through the days . . . wanting to adhere to a schedule, wanting to find some self-discipline, but just too tired and afraid of feeling like crap to do anything.

A small piece of me actually thought I would somehow "get better" and return to work, at least part-time. I was dealing with the guilt of no longer being able to contribute to my family's future. There was also the confusion that came from feeling "better," so should I go back to work? But working made me feel so crappy, and I actually couldn't function. All I could do is sleep.

Then there was the crap about coming to terms with this MS shit. I was probably still in some kind of denial, yet I was so relieved to know that I finally had a legitimate explanation for how crappy this debilitating shit was. I was so totally NOT depressed. As a matter of fact, I think it was actually because I was so psychologically stable that I could sort all this out. There was just so much to mourn, and so much to appreciate the rebirth of.

I wanted to use this time to reinvent myself, and I thought I would in time. I just hadn't been able to do it yet. At fifty years old, I thought my hubby and I would be traveling. I wanted to look for a new job, and I wanted to do more volunteer work at my synagogue. Now, I simply did not have the energy or inclination for any of that, and I was dealing with the new guilt that came from that. Was I "relieved" that I had MS so now I have an excuse to be exempt from those obligations? Or was it because of the MS that I simply could not do these things? Which came first, the chicken or the egg?

After about two months on FMLA, I started to feel something stirring in me. I felt the beginning inklings of peace and acceptance. I knew it was laying somewhere deep down inside. It would come up and find its place in time. I had lots of time, you know. I was never in a rush anymore.

CHAPTER FOURTEEN
MICHELLE

After some time with trying to come to terms with Mom's diagnosis, I decided I could think of it in two ways.

On the one hand, it was so unfair that she was often too tired to do the things I wanted to do together. I couldn't believe she wanted to take a nap instead of coming to Target with me.

On the other hand, I sometimes wondered if her MS was actually a blessing in disguise. Even though it took away a huge part of Mom, it allowed me to see all the good that was inside of her and appreciate her more than I would have if she were healthy. Maybe her MS made our relationship stronger.

I knew she wanted to hide the sickness in her life from me, but she couldn't. Day by day, I watched the disease take control of her life. There was no way she could hide it from any of us. I held out hope that maybe she would learn how to fight the disease, like all of the commercials featuring patients were telling her to do. At the time, though, I thought she was doing a pretty damn good job living her life one day at a time.

Although she was no longer working, I remembered what she had been like when I watched her at work on one of her last days. I'd had an eye appointment, so I got to watch her work while I waited in the lobby. As I watched her move constantly around the displays of eyewear, I knew she wouldn't be working for much longer. She was the happiest miserable person I knew. I watched her interact with her patients, and how she didn't even give a clue that she was sick. She may have had a cane, but she never brought attention toward it. She pretended like it wasn't even there. Like she wasn't even sick.

She was my hero. She was my reality check when I thought my life was too complicated to process. She put everything in the world into perspective for me. The things that *mattered* and the crap that didn't were suddenly so obvious. When I saw all the tiny challenges that Mom was dealing with on a daily basis, I knew I could deal with anything, too. She inspired me to live life while I could and to let go of the little things that didn't matter. In the grand scheme of things, the little shit didn't matter. *Life's short—eat a cookie! Keep it simple, stupid!* She didn't mean to, but she changed my entire perspective on my young adult life. Her experience had somehow made me wise beyond my years.

As the months passed by, she was approved to try new drugs on top of the ones she was already taking, and they had a really high possibility of making her be able to walk again.

"I was approved to try a new drug!" Mom would cry in delight.

"That's so exciting!" my family would respond, enthralled with the feeling of hope.

"You know, if it can just make it so I can walk again, I'll be happy. All I want to do is walk our dog around the block!" she shouted, as Honeybee, our five-year-old boxer-cross, perked up her ears at the word *walk*.

"I just want to take my grandkids to Disney someday," she confessed. "Is that really too much to ask?"

"No," we would reply. "Don't worry, this drug will work!" we constantly reassured her.

A few weeks would go by on the new medication with no real improvements in her abilities. *That was okay*, we thought. We would just try another drug. Try, fail, pick yourself back up, try again. The cycle kept repeating itself.

One of the first drugs she tried was Betaseron. It was given in the form of an injection and delivered in different spots of her body every other day. It was supposed to slow or stop her progression and minimize her attacks.

I had promised that I would support her every way I knew how. If I didn't know how to support her, I would learn. On the day when my family learned how to inject Betaseron, I was the most terrified I had ever been in my life. The nurse was nice enough, but the whole scene felt eerie, surreal. Were we really sitting in our kitchen with a complete stranger, learning how to inject medicine for a crazy disease into my mother's abdomen?

"You'll need to hold the orange button down for ten seconds to make sure all the medicine goes in," I heard the nurse instruct Mom. Mom did as she was told. The button *clicked* as her face winced.

"Did it hurt?" I asked her sympathetically, as she withdrew the needle from her flesh.

"No!" she answered. "It didn't hurt at all!"

I admired her pain tolerance, but I couldn't ignore the tear that landed softly on her cheek. She was actually crying. And *oh my gosh*, Dad was, too. I hadn't seen Dad cry since my grandmother's funeral. I forced myself to look away from them and reminded myself that *this was actually happening*.

"You know, some people who are taking this medicine have been able to start running again!" the nurse told us optimistically.

"Really?" Mom asked, looking starry-eyed.

"Really," she said.

"That's all I want," Mom admitted softly.

We all got turns practicing with an empty injector, learning the best way to position it against her skin and counting to ten before removing it. Once the nurse felt confident in our abilities, she left us on our own with the medicine and the overbearing feeling of *hope*.

For the first few days after every injection, Mom felt like she had the flu. She couldn't get herself out of bed. By the time she began to feel better, it was time for another injection.

Eventually, after COBRA ran out, her insurance wouldn't cover the Betaseron anymore, and it would cost us $3,000 out of pocket to continue using it. We didn't mind giving it up because we hadn't seen anything positive from it anyway. Instead, she began taking a cheaper alternative called Rebif, and again, we were filled with false hope.

˷˷*˷*˷*˷*

I still remember the first moment when I truly thought about the fact that maybe, just maybe, all of this wasn't okay.

It was about two years after she was officially diagnosed, in 2011. I was at a bar on Main Street with Hannah when we ran into a mutual friend of ours named Matt. I had known Matt since kindergarten. We used to play at each other's houses and have breakfast together before school each morning. He lived on my street growing up, so our moms took turns driving us to school. He remembered Mom really well but hadn't seen her since our high school graduation in 2008.

He casually asked, "How's your mom?" and for some odd reason, for the first time since she had been diagnosed, I felt the urge to tell him the truth. I didn't know why the feeling had never struck me before; I think I just truly believed that she was going to be fine. But suddenly, when I looked at Matt, I was terrified that she wouldn't be. Maybe it was because he was an old friend. Maybe it was because he had known her *before.* Maybe it was because I was finally letting the truth sink in.

I wanted to tell him about how she had fallen into the toilet the week before. How she got stuck because she didn't have the strength to lift herself out of it. How she had to wait for two hours for Dad to come home to her rescue because no one else was at the house.

I wanted to tell him about the handicapped railings Dad had just installed all around our house because she couldn't walk without assistance anymore. How hideous and uninviting they were.

I fought back the tears that started burning in the back of my eyes and imagined what it would be like to tell him about the day prior, when I awoke to the sound of her screaming for help because she was falling. She was in her room, and I couldn't get to her in time to catch her. When I reached her, she was laying awkwardly on the floor with her hair sprayed across her face, and her nightgown hiked up to her chest.

I could have just told him that she wasn't *good*, in the traditional sense, but she was trying all kinds of new medicines, so maybe she would get better. But we hadn't seen any indications that she would.

Then I snapped back to reality and concentrated on his words . . . *How is your mom?* That was the question. It was innocent enough. Time was passing by, and I was standing there like an idiot, my eyes darting from side to side with a fake smile on my face. What could I say to him that wouldn't make him completely regret asking me that question? Did he really want to know the answer?

I examined his face for a moment, noting that his eyes weren't looking at me anymore. He seemed more interested in the conversation happening between the people next to us. He might have been an old friend, but he didn't need to hear the truth.

"She's good," I finally lied. "How's yours?" Because, I decided, it was just easier to say that.

And that was how it went for me, at least in the beginning. Every time someone asked me how she was, my mind raced with flashbacks and truths, but I couldn't say any of them out loud. Who would want to listen to that? *No one.* Did I feel like making people depressed every time they asked? *Absolutely not.*

But I did want people to know the truth—I just couldn't articulate the *whole* truth. I started saying things like, "She's okay, thanks for asking," hoping that by saying *okay* instead of *good,* they would understand there was something wrong, but that I didn't really want to talk about it.

People were always really interested in what she was doing to *fight.* They would ask about what kinds of medications she was taking and ask, "Has she heard of that new one?" They would tell me about a "new" theory (which was really only new to them and was just that . . . a theory.)

You know, they think MS might be tied to eating too many chemicals. Has she tried changing her diet?

I heard that yoga helps! Has she tried yoga?

She should see a physical therapist. That will really help her. Has she seen a physical therapist?

Every time someone gave me that type of unsolicited advice, I did the same exact thing: Smiled. Nodded. Muttered lots of *oohs* and *aahs* and even dropped my jaw every now and then, trying to act completely surprised and excited by their new ideas. But I wasn't.

When someone asked me if Mom did yoga, I would have

loved to tell them that she couldn't even stand anymore and didn't have the energy to get herself off the toilet most days. But if I did, they would tell me about *chair yoga* or something else that made it clear that there just *had* to be a solution somewhere, and we just weren't trying hard enough to find it.

When they told me about a new type of drug, I wanted to say *yes, but that's for Relapsing-remitting MS. Mom doesn't have that kind. There are no drugs for the kind she has.* But this would lead into a discussion of the exact details of her MS and that was never a conversation I wanted to have.

Other times, after I said, "She's okay, thanks," I would watch the person's face twist in sympathy and uncertainty. When they knew *okay* meant *not good*, and there weren't any words out there to comfort me. All I would get was a simple *aw* followed by a brief moment of awkward silence until someone changed the subject. But I did give these people credit— at least they weren't trying to bullshit me.

My whole family followed this same strategy when answering the "how's your mom?" question: avoid eye contact, don't say more than five words, and wait patiently for the subject of the conversation to change.

The problem was that after a while, people started to believe us. They really thought that she was "okay," and we couldn't blame them since we never told them otherwise.

Extended family members started to take it personally when Mom didn't attend family gatherings. They didn't understand her lack of communication—was she ignoring their emails? Why wasn't she responding to their messages on Facebook? Was she mad at them? Why didn't she want to come to the family events?

So there came a time, all at once, when Dad, Alex, Mom, and I all sort of flipped a switch. We were sick of pretending and decided that people deserved to know the truth.

"Well, she fell last week," I'd hear Dad tell my uncle casually on the phone.

"Yeah, it really sucks," Alex told me once. "She's really frickin' sick." The fact that Alex admitted it out loud made the whole thing feel so very *real*. And the look on his face when he said it to me for the first time made me want to cry.

Alex wasn't someone to articulate his emotions with words. Growing up, it was often very hard to figure out exactly what he was thinking and feeling. He was such a closed book. For the first few years after Mom's diagnosis, he never said anything out loud about it. To anyone.

When he finally admitted that our Mom was sick, so casually, out loud, to me, his little sister, my heart broke a little. It broke for Mom, for me, and even for Alex. I knew that the pain must have been buried really deep inside of him if it were strong enough to finally transform itself into words.

I may have been the *little* sister, but I wanted so badly to comfort him. I wanted to protect him the way he had protected me from so many things before in my life. I wanted to make him feel *safe*, the way he had made me feel when interrogated my high school boyfriends and fought off the online bullies in middle school. I wanted to make him feel *better*, the way he did when he assured me that the girls who didn't want to be my friends were "losers anyways" and "probably just jealous." I wanted to *help* him the same way he did when he fixed my broken computer time and time again. Alex had never *not* been able to comfort me. Finally, it felt like this was my chance to comfort him. To make him feel less afraid. And yet, I couldn't think of a single thing that I could do or say to make things better. I couldn't make anyone in my family feel better.

Maybe I had my own List of Things, too.

Mom began first admitting the truth through emails to her closest friends, telling them about how she was always tired and how she wished she had her old life back. *No, I'm not ignoring you, I just haven't had any energy all week,* she would explain.

It felt a little like we were somehow all moving through the stages of grief as a solid unit. We were each alone in our grief, but together in our disappointment. At first, we denied it. As we put all our eggs into the medicine basket, we truly thought she would "fight it." It took us a while to move out of the denial phase and into some kind of acceptance. But once we did, and extended family members started to really understand, things got a little better.

At least, Mom got a lot more flowers. Because, really, what do you send to the lady who mysteriously just can't walk anymore and is tired all the time?

CHAPTER FIFTEEN

TAMMY

I wanted to have a cup of tea with my mother so badly. It had been thirteen years since she had died from complications of her diabetes. My memories of her were reduced to only snapshot memories, but I did remember her ever-present beauty. I knew this because of the photo albums of her childhood in the 1920s that I loved to look through. I remembered a black-and-white photograph I had discovered in our basement when I was a little girl. I had brought it to my mother and asked her to explain it to me. It was a long photo that was rolled up in a cardboard tube. After rolling it out to its full length, my mother explained that it was her third-grade class. When I didn't spot her right away, she pointed herself out to me. She was a real cute little girl. She was chubby, with round cheeks and long brown hair. She had banana curls that reached just past her shoulders. In the photo, her hair was parted on the right side, and she had a small clip on the other.

I later came across professional photos of her that must have been her college graduation pictures. As a young adult, she was absolutely beautiful. The photo had been lightly edited, accentuating her features and making her makeup glow as if she were a porcelain doll. She was seated with her arms crossed in front of her, resting on a table. Her fingernails were beautifully manicured. Her earrings sparkled. I knew they were clip-ons because she didn't get her ears pierced until much later in her life.

I was in high school when she was first admitted to the hospital for troubles with her heart. She ended up visiting the hospital a few times because of her faulty heart. After one of her first few hospital stays, she left with a pacemaker. My father sold medical equipment, and at one point, he sold pacemakers. To our family, my mother's pacemaker wasn't such a traumatic ordeal. My dad knew about it, and we all considered him to be our hero, so we knew she was going to be in good hands.

The diabetes came later. I couldn't remember when the actual diagnosis was made or if there was any sense of diabetes as a death decree. She didn't need to change her eating habits since we already ate relatively healthy. She did love to bake and was quite well known for it. The only thing she did differently after her diagnosis was to decrease the amount of sugar that the recipe called for. She never ate many of her treats; instead, she saved the delicacies for others to enjoy. Perhaps that was her enjoyment—watching others eat her delicious treats.

There were vials of insulin on our refrigerator door. Years later, when I was already a young mother, I came for a visit. It was then, for the first time, that I witnessed her giving herself an injection. By that time, she knew she was sick and would not recover, but I did not see it. She was my *mom*. She was the lady who would sit and talk to me for hours on end, telling me stories and listening to mine. She told me stories about her childhood, like how she grew up in Portland, Maine, and all the Jewish families lived near each other so they could be within walking distance to Shul (temple). Her parents lived at the top of the hill. My grandfather owned a furniture store. My grandmother immigrated from Russia.

But she *was* sick. That I didn't want to see it didn't take away the fact that she was sick. She would tell me how her feet would burn. She could only wear certain shoes that were wide enough, so her feet weren't too cramped. Walking on her feet made them hurt even more, but still, she would get up to cook and bake for us. We would sit at the kitchen table with her stories until they turned into the present. She would cry and tell me what the pain was like. I would tell her to dry her tears and that it didn't matter to me if she was sick. I told her I would push her around in a wheelchair through the mall so we could still go shopping together. She tried to explain her illness to me, but whether I *couldn't* or *wouldn't* see it, I didn't know.

I would often think to myself, *Why doesn't she do something to fix herself?* I wanted her to walk more. She had an exercise bike downstairs. Maybe if she used it more she would get better. One year we bought her a foot massager for Hanukkah. You were supposed to fill the basin with water, and when you turned it on, the bottom of it would vibrate. I noticed that she never used it. I thought, *well, if she just used it maybe it would fix her.* It appeared, on the surface, as if she wasn't even trying to help herself get better. I wished she would do more for herself purely so that she could do more for me. How utterly selfish it was for me to think that way.

My mother loved shoes. Going through her closet was one of my favorite pastimes. I was that kind of kid who wanted to rifle through drawers and closets just to see what was there. I wasn't a snoop— I was just looking for something to do. My mother's closet held all kinds of treasures. On the top shelf, she had two jewelry boxes filled with costume jewelry. There were long strands of beaded necklaces, fancy pins, beaded bracelets, and clip-on earrings. She used to get all dolled up before my sister and I were born.

The top shelf also held her important paperwork, such as birth certificates for my sister and me. At the bottom of the closet on the left-hand side were stacks of shoeboxes. They were filled with the shoes that didn't fit on her shoe rack. I would open each box and look at the shoes, wishing they would fit me. But I was too little, and then they were too small as my feet grew to be bigger than my mother's. There were high heels and moccasins and boat sneakers. I used to stroke the high heels, admiring the smoothness of them. I always put them back carefully, just the way I found them, so she wouldn't know I'd been there.

The apple didn't fall far from the tree because I loved shoes, too. I always said that shoes made the outfit. I wasn't one to go to shoe stores and try a whole bunch on. Rather, I would stand and look at the window displays. Only occasionally would I go ahead and try something on with the intention of buying.

Just as my mother could no longer wear her shoes because of the diabetic neuropathy in her feet and legs, I could no longer wear shoes once my feet swelled due to the MS. *Like mother, like daughter.*

I went through my own shoes shortly after my MS diagnosis. I made one pile to throw away, and another pile to give away. I was still walking, but I knew I would never again wear the shoes I had collected throughout the years. I cried when I said good-bye to my lovely shoes, the same way I cried when I gave away all my running clothes. I said good-bye to that part of myself.

I wondered if that was the way my mother felt when she could no longer wear her lovely shoes. Perhaps my mother cried, too, when she was alone, mourning the loss of the person who would never get to see her grandchildren grow up.

~~*~*~*~*

On the one hand, everything was fine. On the other, I was falling apart. I wanted to stop thinking. I wanted to stop pretending. Sometimes I thought, *nah, I don't have MS.* I saw others who had it so bad and would think *that's not me.* Then I read about MS online and thought, *holy crap . . . that* is *me!*

I struggled to understand what Progressive Relapsing MS meant. From my research, I got the idea that MS only struck sick people. But I was certainly not sick. I had been diagnosed at the healthiest point of my life. Never had I been in such great shape.

I wondered what it meant that I was going to get worse. My research taught me that I should continue doing the things I was used to doing—that if I didn't continue moving my body, I would lose the ability to do so. However, when I did things, I felt worse than when I did nothing. If I sat in my chair all day, I felt great. Was I supposed to do *nothing* so that I wouldn't get worse?

Chris was always the person to take me to my doctors' appointments. My neurologist appointments, which were at the same hospital in Lebanon where I had been diagnosed, were very important to me. They were the ones where I learned about the state of my condition. Every time we visited, it felt a little like returning to the scene of the crime. That hospital would always be the place where that one doctor had completely changed my life forever.

Most of the visits blended together in my memory, but there was one that stuck out over the years.

We parked in a handicapped parking spot located in the front row of the visitor parking lot. Handicapped license plates were one of the few perks of having a chronic disease like MS. I was incredibly thankful for the advocates at the National MS Society, who fought tooth and nail to help people like me have access to handicapped license plates.

As Chris opened my car door and I felt the hot July sun beat down on me, I was instantly thankful for the shortened walk across the parking lot. Chris positioned my walker in front of me and lifted me out of the car.

I walked slowly to the entrance of the hospital, and my husband stayed by my side the entire time, keeping his left hand on the walker as an extra layer of support. I wondered if he was preparing himself to catch me if I were about to fall.

Fortunately, I didn't fall. I made it all the way to the lobby of the waiting room on my own two feet. And then I couldn't walk anymore.

Instead, I sat on the bench of my walker and waited patiently for my name to be called. Chris completed the paperwork, knowing all too well that writing was becoming more and more challenging for me. It was easier for the both of us if he wrote for me.

After a few minutes, my name was called. Chris pushed me on my walker to the cozy room where the doctor would be in shortly to see us.

Moments later, she knocked on the door. My neurologist was a real hot shit. I think Chris actually had a little thing for her. She was of Russian descent and had beautiful, perfect skin and short, blonde hair. Her smile lit up the room, and her positive energy always enthused me. She was down-to-earth and smart. She didn't try to bullshit us, which fueled the amount of respect Chris held for her.

"Hello!" she exclaimed as she entered the room, shaking both of our hands immediately. "How are you doing, Tammy!" She said it as more of an exclamation than a question.

"Hi," Chris and I responded in unison.

"I'm okay," I said. "I don't feel sick all the time anymore, which is nice."

She nodded and smiled, probably feeling grateful for this bit of positive news.

"I just feel like *me* now," I added, before pressing on. "Maybe it's me trapped in a strange body, but as long as I don't do anything, I'm fine."

I thought about the way I had been living for the three months since I had seen her last. I had taken a leave of absence from work and then decided not to return. I learned that I had moments when I felt great and wanted desperately to do a variety of things. But I also learned that when I acted on those impulses and proceeded to do things like cook dinner or straighten the mess on the counter, then I crashed. Sometimes the crash was a real fall. I hated falling.

I told her about this constant imbalance, of wanting to continue feeling great but feeling like I would rather stay busy, even if that meant I would feel horrible later. "Should I do stuff because I can, even though I'll feel like a puddle after? Or should I sit and enjoy feeling good?" I asked her curiously.

She didn't give me a clear answer. "Well, I think it's about listening to your body," she told me. "It's important that you continue using whatever functionality you still have, or else you will lose the ability to do so."

I had heard this before. I called it the *use it or lose it* phenomenon.

She proceeded to tell me about what I might expect in the next few months and asked for an update on the Rebif I had been taking. I told her it was fine, that things were going just fine.

"I don't think I've gotten better," I admitted. "But I haven't gotten worse, either. I'm fine. We're all fine."

My comment was followed by a cold silence. I realized Chris hadn't said anything for a while. *What was he thinking?* I wondered. I truly thought everything and *everyone* were really fine. But his silence and slouched shoulders were telling me otherwise.

I looked closely at his face and noticed a tear on his cheek.

At first, it didn't hit me. I didn't really think much of it. I looked at him and thought *oh, gee. He's kind of crying.*

I didn't think, *What's he sad about?* I just made the observation and didn't think anything else of it. I didn't even bother to call attention to it or ask him what was wrong. I just thought it was

How's Your Mom?

odd. Why was he crying about me?

My neurologist didn't call attention to it, either. She just kept talking, informing us of what our future might look like. She kept saying things like "You might not always feel worse, but you are progressively getting worse."

I wondered what that meant. I didn't feel worse. I just felt like me. I guessed this was what my friend, Leslie, who also had MS, was talking about when she talked about what's "normal." It was normal now to walk . . . *hmm, walk?* I might be using that term loosely. It was normal to *lean/walk* on the left side of a hallway now so I could crawl along the wall. It was normal now to not even try to carry anything. It was normal to know all my grab spots in the house. It was normal to get out of a sitting position by pushing up with my arms. It was normal to ask for help and accept an out-stretched hand.

I wasn't getting *worse*. I was getting *smart*! I was so proud of every way I've figured out to help me get around! I was so smart! I was still me!

I was so comfortable! I loved my iPad! I loved when Alex sat and watched TV with me. I loved when Michelle called to talk to me.

I was me. I was not MS.

CHAPTER SIXTEEN

MICHELLE

Not every day was a bad day. She had a lot of really good days that were mixed in with the rough ones. On a really good day, we could have hours together before her body quit on her.

In the middle of March 2010, Mom and I went to Panera for lunch. We each ordered a smoothie, mine with a turkey sandwich and hers with a salad. After a lovely lunch, we wanted to go to Kohl's. Almost immediately upon walking into Kohl's, we both figured out that the smoothies from Panera must have had laxatives! Mom and I weren't ones to talk about our bodily functions (we were both far too ladylike for that), but it seemed that the smoothies had the same undeniable effect on both of us. Laughing, we both made it to the bathroom on time.

We made our way back to the racks of clothes and began searching for a new purse for her. It needed to be small because she couldn't carry a regular-sized purse anymore. It was too heavy. We found an adorable, solid black Vera Wang wristlet, and confirmed that the essential accessories could all fit inside: Chapstick, a couple of credit cards, license, tissues, and keys. There wasn't a ton of extra room or weight . . . it was perfect.

The clutch was really cute; it was the first accessory of hers I found myself actually approving, which was weird because I thought she'd told me that she majored in fashion in college. Yet I had never *once* been envious of her fashion choices until she bought that black clutch. I wanted to borrow that clutch.

We browsed through the clothing racks, and she agreed to buy me a new white sweater. As I took one off the rack with the intention of trying it on over my t-shirt, I accidentally interrupted a middle-aged woman who was also reaching for an item on the same rack.

"Oh, sorry," I mumbled at her as I snatched my hand back like I had been shocked.

She didn't respond. Instead, she shot me a look of pure disapproval. I could read her mind: *What an oblivious young girl. How dare she get in my way. Those Millennials are so entitled!* I continued looking at her, waiting for her to respond, to tell me it was okay, or that she forgave me.

She looked back at me, her dirty look becoming even dirtier by the millisecond. Truthfully, I was a little bit afraid. I retracted my gaze, focusing instead on the floor in front of me.

Mom glared back at her, completely baffled by the entire exchange. When the woman finally walked away, I turned to look at Mom. "What was her problem?"

"She's a grouch," she told me. "She's probably either really constipated or in need of a good orgasm."

I scoffed loudly and immediately turned away from Mom. *Oh my G-d! An orgasm? Was I hearing her correctly?* I was nineteen years old, and Mom was helping me understand that some people became grouchy because they needed to have sex. What kind of mom said those things to her teenaged daughter?

I laughed and blushed, still too immature to be able to continue the conversation, but grateful that I had such a realistic, transparent mom.

After Kohl's, we went to a paint-your-own-pottery place. She made me a wine goblet and decorated it with the colors of the college I was attending. She wrote, "Keene 2012" (my year of graduation) and "I Hope You Dance" on the sides. I made her a water mug, wrote, "I love you," and used stencils to draw pretty flowers on the sides.

Next, we went to the Hallmark store to pick up some cards. As we stood in the silent aisle, browsing through every single card (because you can't buy one before you read them all), she let out the loudest, squeakiest fart I had ever heard. I swear it went on for ten seconds. She couldn't make it stop! We both blushed in embarrassment and even apologized to the girl who had been stocking cards in the aisle next to us. She told us she didn't hear it, but we knew that was impossible. She absolutely heard it. We laughed about that fart for at least half an hour. I didn't think I could ever love my mom more than I did at that moment.

Amazingly, we continued our journey to Rite Aid. "Mom, do you want to take a basket? Don't we need a lot of stuff?" I asked her.

She shook her head and continued dragging her legs toward the toothpaste aisle. She was using a cane at this point, and she leaned heavily on it now. She was doing fine, so I shrugged and walked toward the shampoo.

I was still debating which brand of shampoo to buy when I heard a loud *CRASH* come from a few aisles over. *Oh, no,* I thought to myself. *Please don't let that be Mom.*

I hurried to the most embarrassing aisle in the store, otherwise known as the incontinence aisle, and found Mom surrounded by a variety of items scattered around the floor. Adult diapers, pads, toothpaste, Metamucil, Preparation H, and dental floss stared up at her from the floor. She stared back at them, not even attempting to pick them up. She spotted me, watching her, and immediately burst into a fit of laughter.

Her laughter was contagious, and instead of immediately picking everything up, we both just stood there, laughing. I shook my head at her and continued laughing until we both caught our breath.

I walked away from her, toward the baskets that we walked by earlier, and picked one up. I brought it back to the embarrassing aisle and picked up her huge mess. Her smile didn't fade as she watched me work.

I carried her basket to the checkout aisle, then carried her bags to the car.

When we finally arrived home, Mom sang, "Home again, home again, jiggity jig!" I rolled my eyes, the way I always did when she said that stupid phrase.

I couldn't help but give the Rebif all of the credit for our day. It must have been helping. Five months before, she wouldn't have lasted for four hours like she had. She could even walk a few steps without her cane. I thought, again, about how she was my hero.

Little did I know, it would be the last time we would ever

go shopping together.

*_*_*_*_*_*

August 25, 2010
Dear Michelle,

Summer is coming to an end, and this weekend you will go back to Keene State College for your third year. We have not shared too much these past few months. Is it because there is nothing worth discussing? Or because we are just letting life happen right now?

I feel so close to you right now that I think we just talk about whatever we want when we are face-to-face. We don't need the pen to aid us in sharing.

I am forever appreciative and grateful to have you in my life. But I have to mark today's event so we will always remember it.

This is the evening you went out for ice cream with Hannah, and you backed your car into Alex's in our driveway. You left quite a good dent in both of your cars. I wonder how, years from now, the story will be told. I know we will laugh, but I wonder how brother and sister will grow from this experience.

Of course, I feel guilty. If only I had backed my car in, parked on the other side, warned you about where Alex's car was parked. But alas, the shoulda, woulda, couldas *fix nothing.*

And so I just wonder. I care so little about the material objects and treasure my family, our life and our relationships so dearly. It tires me sometimes to be the thread to hold us all together. I try so hard. When something unravels, I feel so helpless. And so, I will let life happen . . .

I feel I should be offering some great words of wisdom from which you will find comfort and think, wow—my mom knows exactly what to say to make everything right! *But all I can think is* shit happens! *All I can say is I love you so much, no matter what.*

You cry, I laugh, Alex hides. Bubbie would say all you have is each other.

Life—your life, my life, Alex's life, Dad's life—goes on. We remain our little family with our little Honeybee dog.

I love you more than words can say and forever.

I hope you dance,

CHAPTER SEVENTEEN

MICHELLE

How was it possible that day by day nothing seemed to change, but when I looked back, everything was different? As each day passed, there were no indications, at least from my perspective, that her disease was progressing. Sometimes she was more tired than other days, but wasn't that the case for all of us?

Life carried on around us. I worked a lot and Dad spent a ton of time working from the basement. Mom seemed sad a lot, so I did everything I could to try to cheer her up. I'd offer ideas for things we could do together, places we could go and shows we could see. One time I even went so far as to score handicapped-accessible seats at an Adele concert, thinking that if I already had them in my online shopping cart, then she would have no choice but to say, *what a great idea! You've thought of everything! Of course, I'll go with you!* But instead, she told me that getting to a concert would be too hard. She apologized, although she didn't have to, and told me she would have loved to go *if she could.*

I struggled to understand what she meant by "if she could." Was she saying that she really couldn't go? Why? I mean, I had gotten handicapped-accessible seats. People with walkers went to concerts ALL THE TIME. We could even put her in a wheelchair for the day to make things easier. It wasn't a big deal. Why did she insist on putting these limits on herself? Why did she get always get to decide what we were allowed to do?

The only ideas I had about things we could do that she seemed to genuinely be excited about were the activities that I could *do,* and she could *watch.*

"Hey, Mom, want to make cookies?" I'd ask her.

"Sure, I'll come watch you and tell you what to do," she would reply.

"Hey, Mom, want to help me organize these pictures?"

"Sure, I'll tell you where to put them."

"Hey, Mom, can you show me how I should iron this shirt?"

"Sure, I'll tell you what to do."

Sure . . . she'd tell. She'd watch. She'd be there. But she wouldn't be able to participate.

After a while, I could tell she was starting to feel like a fly on the wall. Even at the dinner table, I noticed her participating in our conversations less and less. Was it because she wasn't interested? Were we talking too fast for her to be able to jump in? Or did she just wish she were taking a nap instead of sitting there with us?

I had so many questions. Nothing about our life with the villain made sense. And yet, we all carried on as if everything was fine. What other choice did we have?

One particularly "fine" morning, it was just Mom and I in the house. Dad wasn't home, and Alex had already moved out into his own home. It was 2012, and I had graduated from college and moved back in with my parents, trying to get my foot in the door of a real career before I had to start paying off my student loans.

I was sound asleep when I was woken up by the sound of my cell phone ringing loudly in my ear. I was livid that someone would be calling me at the extremely early hour of nine a.m., but I checked the caller ID anyway. It was Mom. Her bedroom was on the first floor and mine was on the second, and she couldn't yell loud enough for me to hear her. So I had told her to call me in the event of any emergency.

Even though I had only just awoken, my heart started to race, and I got that feeling that you get when you wake up from a terrible dream.

With shaky hands, I answered the phone with a quick "hi," and waited for her response.

She was crying, and her voice was choppy, but she managed to ask, "Can you come help me?"

I didn't even bother answering. I hung up the phone and flew out of bed. I ran as fast as a person can when they're still half-asleep and trying not to fall down the stairs.

When I finally reached her room, I saw that she was still in bed. That was a good sign because it meant that she hadn't fallen or hurt herself, so there was no immediate danger.

"What's wrong?" I asked, suddenly annoyed that she woke me up but still curious as to why she needed my help. She was lying on her side, her face was drenched in tears, but she appeared unharmed.

"I can't move," she sobbed out to me. "I have to pee, I can't move, and I think I'm going to pee the bed."

And just like that, I was awake. I needed to think fast. First things first, I needed to figure out the fastest way to pick her up out of bed. She was lying awkwardly on her side, so I needed to sit her up straight before I could pick her up. As I tried to move her legs, so they faced the outside of the bed, I quickly discovered that they were solid. They wouldn't bend. It was like they were made of stone. I was so baffled by her legs that I momentarily forgot what I was doing and lost track of the fact that she might pee her bed.

That's okay, I decided. Her legs didn't really need to bend. After a short struggle with the blankets and her heavy legs, I managed to get her to an upright position. She sat on the edge of the bed with her legs sticking straight out. How awkward. I needed to basically straddle her to pick her up out of bed. This was going to be super fun.

Her walker was positioned behind me as I prepared to pick her up. She only weighed about a hundred pounds, but my hands were trembling, and I was supporting her entire weight. I needed to get her to sit down on the walker, but it was behind me, and I needed to turn her around first.

I forgot that her legs were sticking out straight, so as I tried to turn her around, her leg caught on the side of the bed, and I lost my balance. All at once I began falling toward the bed, still trying to support Mom but thinking about how we were both going to fall to the ground. I was holding her so awkwardly that I couldn't balance her correctly.

I panicked.

The side of my torso caught the edge of the bed. I grabbed onto the edge with my free arm, and it stopped us from crashing

How's Your Mom?

down.

Finally, I managed to get her balanced and into her walker. I rolled her to the bathroom as fast as I could. She explained that if she peed it wouldn't be that hard to clean up, and that she'd help me. The word "help" rang loudly in my head, knowing all too well this meant she would *tell* me what to do, but not actually *help*.

We finally made it to the bathroom when we encountered our next problem. Her legs were still sticking out straight, and I couldn't maneuver her around the laundry hamper that had officially gotten in our way. We were about two feet from the toilet, but we were stuck, and I didn't know what to do. I was trying so hard to bend her legs, to no avail. "WHAT THE HELL!" I screamed out loud.

Meanwhile, she was still crying and obviously trying extremely hard not to pee her pants.

I re-adjusted the laundry hamper by chucking it across the bathroom floor, causing the dirty clothes to spray all around the bathroom. I didn't care. I had finally gotten her in the proper position to use the toilet. "Okay, Mom, we're there," I told her.

"Are you sure?" she asked.

"Yes," I responded back, and I stared at her. Suddenly, I was horrified. "Am I going to have to take your underwear off?" I was absolutely mortified.

"I'm so, so sorry," she cried to me slowly, each word sounding more broken than the last. I couldn't bring myself to respond.

I pulled her underwear down and told her it was okay for her to sit. She stayed where she was, squatting awkwardly over the toilet, looking extremely uncomfortable.

"SIT!" I yelled at her.

She looked at me, blinked back another tear, and stayed crouching an inch above the toilet seat.

"MOM! SIT!" I didn't get it. Why wouldn't she sit?

Suddenly she started peeing. *Good for her*, I thought silently to myself. Still, I held her side to make sure she didn't fall over.

Her legs were still hard as stone. I stayed silent because the sound of her peeing made me unable to speak. It was too awkward.

This couldn't be happening.

"It's called muscle rigidity," she informed me.

Sweet, I thought. *I was hoping I'd get to learn about that today.*

When she finally finished her business, she explained to me that she'd slept too long without taking her muscle relaxer, and that was her consequence. I asked what pills she needed to take and brought the medicine to her. I twisted the cap off for her, handed her two pills and she took swallowed them dry. I let her sit on the toilet for a couple minutes until the medicine kicked in. I somehow managed not to cry, but she hadn't stopped. I wished there was something I could say, do, ask . . . but I had nothing.

After about five minutes I picked her up off the toilet, placed her in the white wicker chair in her bedroom and made her some coffee. She was better then, so I knew it was safe for me to go back upstairs.

As I walked back upstairs, I wondered to myself what the hell had just happened and tried desperately to erase the whole thing from my memory.

CHAPTER EIGHTEEN

TAMMY

Progressive MS was just that— progressive.

The weakness in my left side continued as my left hand became more useless. I went from being able to hold something in my left hand and manipulate a knife with my right, to the left being no help at all. What would happen when my right hand no longer functions either?

The vibrating that was once only in my left leg progressed to my right leg. I finally got an electric wheelchair, which was a huge help. It had a logo printed on it that said "Jazzy Blue," so this is what we called it. My Jazzy Blue chair. As promised, it got me from one spot to another to help conserve some energy.

The days blended into each other. The weeks rolled along. The sameness of the days was both comforting and unnerving. I mourned the loss of my once so-busy life. I was so busy. I missed the days when I could just jump up and run off to the store and do an errand.

When I said I didn't feel good, what exactly did I mean? It was a headache. A bit of nausea. That feeling of having to poop. I felt like my glasses were crooked. Was I dizzy, off balance, seeing double? No. Not always. It was all just not right. I couldn't hold my head up. I couldn't hold my body up. I was lightheaded like I needed some water, or juice, or a cookie. Only none of that made it go away. Only sleep helped me to escape.

Every May, Chris took his yearly trip to Montana. This year, Michelle was in charge of taking care of me. Every day, I couldn't stop myself from thinking, *Wow. She's amazing, and I am so very lucky to have her.* There simply weren't enough words to express my love and gratitude for my princess.

But it was so frustrating that she had to see me that way. I tried so hard to be strong. At times, I could muster some strength. Other times, I needed to call for help.

One night, I was lying in bed, and I simply could not

move. My legs were frozen. My arms were weak. There was some strength, so it's not like I was paralyzed, but I needed help. The first wave of reality came when I had to pee, but could not move. I had to call Michelle.

She got me up and was shocked by the rigidity in my legs. She got me to the toilet in time.

It's not such a great thing to pee while your daughter keeps you upright. It's not something a daughter should have to do.

After that, I didn't make it to the toilet on time twice. I did make it to the bathroom floor, rather than the rug, but it was demoralizing nonetheless. I hated for Michelle to see me like that.

I still held a secret wish for a miraculous cure. I still dreamed about walking. I still thought about what kind of job I'd like to get, and what I would bake and cook for my family when that miracle cure happened. But mostly, my story had come to be one of calm and comfort. Being a naturally passive person, it was not too difficult for me to surrender to the proverbial riptide. The support I received from my family was instrumental. My husband took care of everything from housework to paying bills, from getting me coffee to getting me showered. My daughter babysat me often. My son kept all my computer and Internet devices working. So my story became focused on how to not become a negative bitch. Moments centered around appreciation and gratitude, which was hard because I used to be the main caretaker and do-er.

I used to be *the mom*. It was a role I cherished and tried so hard to be good at. The role reversal stood stark as my daughter was the one to leave for work each morning while I stayed home.

My story would continue as the disability progressed. Yes, I was scared. But I was safe, and I was blessed.

I knew I must enter this new life. Yet I still resisted. Why?

How's Your Mom?

CHAPTER NINETEEN

MICHELLE

After that whole stone-leg incident took place, I decided to avoid Mom for a while. It was pretty easy, honestly, because she began receiving chemotherapy treatments, and those knocked her out *cold* for at least five days. We had been told that if she received chemotherapy, her disease might stop progressing. It seemed, for a while, like the Rebif was actually helping, but it wasn't. She was still getting worse. So we decided we would give chemotherapy a shot. Why not? What did we have to lose? We knew it wouldn't make her better, but we were (once again) filled with the hope that she wouldn't get worse.

However, for the days after she received treatment, she couldn't even get out of bed. Her chemotherapy took whatever little energy she had and spent it. For that reason (and a million others), she wondered what the point of it was. It was hard to continue receiving treatment when the benefit wasn't immediately apparent. It was harder to receive it when we felt like she was still getting worse. She only ended up receiving chemotherapy treatments for a few months before she finally gave up on those, too.

After about a week of ignoring her, I found her seated in her cozy chair in the living room. I still wanted to avoid her. The more I did, the easier it was for me to pretend like everything was okay. But it had been a full week since the pee incident, and seeing her sitting in her chair looking so bored and lonely made something inside of me ache. I knew she didn't deserve my coldness. I knew none of this was her fault. It wasn't her fault that she couldn't do things with me like she used to. It wasn't her fault that she was tired all the time. But if I couldn't blame her, who could I blame?

I decided that I should suck it up and sit with her. Before I did, I scooped myself a bowl of ice cream and gave myself a mental pep talk. I swore to myself that I would just listen. I swore I would be patient and receptive to whatever she wanted to talk about. I swore I would be respectful.

As I walked toward the living room, I could practically feel her mood brighten. It was as if I were a ray of sunshine that was melting her icy MS core.

Since it had been an entire week, I thought she was going to have a lot to say. I started eating my ice cream, and, as expected, she immediately engaged me in conversation. She told me about her latest dose of chemotherapy and complained about how Dad bought the wrong kind of yogurt at the grocery store. She asked how my friends were doing and listened intently as I told her what a few of them had been up to.

Once she had exhausted all of her small talk topics, she asked me if I knew who Annette Funicello was. I had never heard of her. "No," I said shortly.

"Annette used to be a part of this group called The Mouseketeers," she explained. I had never heard of the group. "They were really popular when I was growing up." I sensed that she was about to tell me a story that was somehow related to Annette, and I honestly wasn't at *all* interested in hearing it. But I remembered the pep talk I had given myself just minutes ago and forced myself to repeat it in my head: *Be patient. Listen to her. Be respectful.*

"You know, I subscribe to that blog called *The Wheelchair Kamikaze,*" she told me.

I thought for a moment, recalling what I knew about *The Wheelchair Kamikaze.* Mom talked about it *all the time.* It was her favorite MS blog. For that reason, I had read it a few times myself, but I didn't subscribe to it like Mom did. From what I could tell, it was a funny, informational, honest blog written by a man named Marc who had MS. "I know," I said.

Apparently, my saying "I know," did not satisfy her enough. She must have thought I needed more back story about the blog. "He's really honest, you know," she continued.

"I know," I repeated again, a sharp edge to my tone.

"And he's really smart, and he writes about a lot of the current events happening with MS research and stuff," Mom blabbed on. I already knew *all* of this. But in the spirit of not being rude, I let her speak, and in turn, increasingly lost interest in the conversation. Still, I sat there, eating my ice cream and choosing to avoid eye contact. *Be patient. Listen to her. Be respectful.* It was like a mantra I had to keep repeating.

"*The Wheelchair Kamikaze* posted an article about Annette," she began to explain. "She was diagnosed with MS a while ago and has been very quiet ever since."

She at least had spiked my attention, but I still wasn't sure where she was going with this story. A few moments passed, and still, I sat there, curious and confused, unable to ask any kind of follow-up question.

"The media never focuses on the people who have the bad kind of MS," she started again. "You only hear about the people who have the good kind of MS." *Yeah, like Ann Romney,* I thought to myself. *Or that hockey player who still plays hockey. What was his name? Tyler would know.* There was a pause, and then she said under her breath, "You never hear about the people like me."

It was true. You didn't. Her disease was too sad to talk about out loud.

I stayed quiet while she continued to describe the blog post. To be honest, I still wasn't sure where this story was going, and my *pretend to give a damn* was running pretty low. I realized I was almost done with my bowl of ice cream, and I hoped her story would end soon so I could go back to the kitchen and get more.

Instead, she continued. "Well, the introduction of the blog entry warns you that what proceeds is a description of the really bad stuff that can result from MS. It shows what happened to Annette. It says you should stop reading if you think it will be disturbing."

She paused long enough for me to realize that it was my turn to talk. I opened my mouth, but nothing came out. I wasn't sure what to say.

I stuttered for a bit, then, still afraid of where the conversation was going, blurted, "Well, did you read it?" My tone completely blew the whole *don't be rude* thing.

If she thought my tone was snappy, she didn't let on. She just answered the question. "No, not yet."

Phew, I thought. *Maybe this wouldn't be so bad.*

But she continued. "I'm going to read it tomorrow, so I don't have nightmares tonight. But I've heard what happened to Annette."

There was a pause again. This time it felt like all of the air had been sucked out of our cozy living room. The silence seemed to drag on forever. I didn't want to know what happened to Annette. *Please don't tell me, please don't tell me, please don't tell me. . . .*

And just like that, she dropped the bomb. "She can't swallow anymore."

Damn it. *Damn it, damn it, damn it.* Why did she tell me that? Why?

Ironically, I lost the ability to swallow at that moment as well. I began swirling my remaining spoonful of ice cream around in the bowl. What could I say to that?

"How does that happen?" I asked her. I realized immediately after the words escaped that the question was rhetorical and completely ridiculous, but it was all I could come up with.

As any good mom would, she tried to provide an answer for her seemingly curious daughter. "Well, MS controls your nerves. There are nerves that make you swallow, and when you lose those . . ." Her voice trailed off as I fought the urge to scream, *YES, MOM. I GET IT. THANK YOU.*

A few moments passed before I finally thought of something better to say. "Well, that's not going to happen to you!" I told her. As I said it, I felt myself sit up a little straighter and heard my voice jump an octave. I tried to sound positive, but while I was speaking I could feel my body start to shake, my teeth begin to chatter, and I couldn't for the life of me force my eyes to meet hers. Was I lying? I really didn't think I was.

"It probably will," she told me, and suddenly that bomb exploded.

That was it. At this point, I was angry. Furious. Livid. So I did what I always did when these feelings struck: I snapped back into my place of denial. It was the comforting spot in my head where I could hide and pretend like everything's fine.

"But that's why you're doing chemo," I reminded her, a

little too aggressively. "It's going to slow your progression and make it so you don't get worse."

"Chemo is only for a little while. It doesn't make me better. I'm never going to be the way I used to be," she said. "It's funny . . . I used to really believe that one day I'd get better. I used to practice using my hand and tell myself that I would eventually get it to work again."

I was numb. Numb to it all. "You can still get better," I eventually stuttered, staring at the coffee table in front of me. Yet even in my state of denial, I knew I was lying.

"I'm just delaying the inevitable," she told me. A few silent moments passed by. It felt like an eternity passed before she spoke again. "Thanks for listening. I'm just rambling."

I nodded and tried to wait as long as possible before leaving the room. After twenty seconds or so, I couldn't stand it any longer. I needed to escape. With shaky legs and an aching heart, I walked up the stairs to my bedroom as normally as possible.

I reached the top of the stairs, stepped into my bedroom and slowly closed my door. I collapsed on my bed, put my head in my hands and imagined what it would be like to have a mother who couldn't swallow anymore. A mother who needed to use a feeding tube to get essential nutrients. A mother who couldn't enjoy birthday cake anymore.

The whole thing was too much for me to comprehend, so I retreated back to my state of denial because it was nicer there and I liked it better. Instead of letting the tears fall from my eyes, I decided to be strong and go back downstairs. I scooped myself another bowl of ice cream and made lots of noise, so Mom knew I was downstairs, not just hiding in my room. I wanted her to think I was fine. I wanted everyone to think I was fine. And after I finished demonstrating just how *fine* I was, I crept silently back upstairs to my room and thought about the fact that maybe I really was *not* fine.

CHAPTER TWENTY

TAMMY

It came on like a wave. The warning was in the white-caps that slowly rose and taunted me. I knew it was coming, but I couldn't run from it. It rose up. My vision went wonky. It crested. My body folded over. It crashed down. I couldn't move. Why? Something I ate? Something I did? The heat? The stress? Fatigue?

There was no common denominator. What brought it on one day did not the next.

It was like a washcloth. At first, it was dry and stiff. Water slowly dampened it. It became limp as it saturated. The water began to leak out until a puddle formed. I would wring the washcloth out. I squeezed and twisted it until it was no longer dripping. I could start again.

The tears built up in an emotional response to the loss . . . of function, of control, of desire. I willed my body to cooperate, but tears poured out instead.

In my mind, I saw a need to do something. In my mind, I made a plan. It was such a simple task: *Move the cup from one spot to another. Fill it with water. Hold the cup. Bring it to my mouth. Tilt my head back. Swallow.* All while standing? That was too much. Too frustrating.

It was a physical response to the mixed-up energy sent out by the mixed-up nerves. The nerves needed to rest. They needed to weep. The tears needed to wash away the feeling.

So I slept . . . and it passed.

CHAPTER TWENTY-ONE

CHRIS

I liked to think that for the first twenty-five years of our marriage, my wife took care of me. She cooked our family dinner every night, made sure the house was always clean and gave me space to pursue my hobbies, to do my own thing. Some of my favorite hobbies are owning guns, shooting my guns, cleaning my guns, and selling my old guns so I could buy new guns. Every year, my buddies and I liked to take a trip out to Montana where we could shoot all of our guns.

A lot of people used to ask her why she "let me" go to Montana every year. As if I needed permission. (Okay, maybe I did.) But when people asked her this, she'd throw her head back and laugh. "*Let him?*" she'd reply. "I don't *let* him do anything! He does whatever he wants!"

Maybe this was why we had stayed married for over thirty years. She didn't try to control me. Not once. She *let* me do whatever I wanted. And going to Montana every year was something I really wanted to do.

And yeah, she took great care of me. She loved our kids and put them above everything else in our life. We had a simple life, but we liked it that way. We were happy.

When her foot started to drag, I didn't mind giving her a shoulder to lean on. I let her lean on me when she got tired and just needed a break. When she couldn't lift her foot to walk up the stairs, I would pick it up and put it on the next step for her. I drove her to doctor's appointments all around New England, trying to make sure I was living up to my promise of *taking care of her*. Once she stopped being able to walk, I left the company where I was working so I could stay at home all day and be with her, just in case she needed someone. She always said she would be fine all alone, but once she started falling, I wouldn't have her left alone anymore.

It was what it was. Her disability became part of our life, our routine. She stopped being able to cook and clean, so I started doing it. (Well, I started trying to learn how to cook. I really only like chicken, so that's mostly what I made. If no one else wanted to eat it, they could go to hell.)

My children tried to help out whenever they could. We were so lucky to have them; they were good kids. But Tammy never wanted them to have to be a part of her disease. She never wanted them to have to see her become so sick.

As the years went by, Tammy needed a growing amount of supervision. I never wanted her to be left alone. Once both of our kids moved out, I was the only one really taking care of her. It was a full-time job. I didn't mind, though. She was my wife, and I loved her. Plus, I promised I'd do it. A real man never breaks his promises.

Sometimes, though, the sadness of it all did creep up on me. I didn't ever want to admit how sad I was. I wasn't the kind of man to cry. It wasn't the way I'd been raised. But I did need a break sometimes, and that's when my trips to Montana became even more important.

My other favorite hobby was my car. I'm a classic car guy. For a few years, I had been the proud owner of a 1970 Chevelle SS. It was painted a nice, shiny red, with black racing stripes on the hood. Whenever anything broke on it, I'd fix it. I drove it around town and took it to car shows in the summertime. I had a group of car buddy friends with whom I hung out at the car shows.

At the car shows, I'd display a fake, stuffed parrot on the car. I'd perch it right in the center of the hood, and when people walked by, it would squawk *hey, go fuck yourself!* It made me laugh every time. Some people thought it was absolutely obscene, and every now and then it would squawk at a kid, which maybe wasn't a great look for me. That, accompanied by the fake stuffed child I put under the tire, might have made me look like a psychopath. There might have been something wrong with me. Maybe I had a few screws loose.

I didn't care. I thought it was hilarious. It was so much fun. It was a distraction from my real life.

How's Your Mom?

CHAPTER TWENTY-TWO

TAMMY

In his sleep, he frowned. The worry line between his brows furrowed more and more deeply. He snored a *purr*-like sound. He asked why I "let" him do what he wants? Why did I let him go play with his red car and go to car shows?

Because when he was in his red car, he had fun. He laughed and forgot all his worries.

He always came home to me.

--*-*-*-*-*

My life had become one big contradiction.

I was supposed to be grateful. Grateful that it wasn't worse. Grateful that I wasn't dying. Grateful that it wasn't cancer or some other horrible disease. Grateful that I had a wonderful, caring, understanding family. Grateful that I had a comfortable home and I was safe. Grateful that I had plenty of food. Grateful that I had the companionship of a loyal dog. Grateful to the friends who wanted to come visit me. The list went on and on.

I was grateful. At least, I was grateful enough to acknowledge it all. But how was all of this *gratefulness* going to help me?

I said *please, thank you,* and *I'm sorry.* But I didn't get better. I didn't get happier. I didn't make other people better.

Instead of being grateful, I wished I would die. After all, what kind of life was I actually living? I didn't get to go skydiving or Rocky Mountain climbing, like the guy in Tim McGraw's song, "Live Like You Were Dying." I didn't get to go "two point seven seconds on a bull named Fu Manchu." It all just slowly disappeared. Instead of getting better, I faded away.

I had to witness my family watch the slow decline in my ability to function. I wanted to hide my struggles, but I wanted them to know the truth, too. They watched me, and I wondered what they must think. Were they angry for all that they, too, missed out on?

I was the kind of mom who always wanted to be there for

my kids. I helped them shop for their events and prepare for their next milestones. And my hubby and I were going to travel. We would only be fifty years old when our children would be grown and independent.

Food became a struggle, too. I didn't want to eat too many calories because gaining weight would make it even more difficult to drag this body around. It would have made it harder for Chris to pick me up.

I used to say *life is short, eat a cookie!* The problem was . . . it wasn't short. It was dragging on, and the joys of eating cookies were replaced with the reality of weight gain.

The work of meal preparation was huge. Even a simple meal of veggies required standing and assembling. It wasn't even safe for me to use a knife or the stove. I could not reach into the oven.

My beautiful home held me captive. The fear of venturing too far from my safety zone was overwhelming. At home, I had my routine. I could nap.

Before I was diagnosed, when I was so ridiculously tired every morning, and I left my bedroom, I would glance back at my bed and say good-bye to it. I would murmur *I'll be back soon, comfy bed.* At the same time, something deep inside of me said, *be careful what you wish for. Someday you will be bedridden.*

CHAPTER TWENTY-THREE
MICHELLE

I really didn't know anything. I didn't know how I was supposed to handle conversations like the one Mom and I had about what the future of her MS might look like, and about people like Annette Funicello. Did she like talking to me about her disease? Did I come across as rude during those conversations? Did she dread having to tell me things like that? Or was it part of her plan, as my mother, to have those types of conversations to prepare me for whatever was to come?

Growing up, I could tell Mom anything, and it was absolutely great. I felt so lucky to have such a close relationship with her where I felt comfortable sharing everything with her.

But as her disease progressed, it felt like the tables had turned. I didn't want to tell her anything because my problems seemed tiny and pathetic compared to hers. Yet she still wanted to share things with me. It was so sad that I really didn't want to listen. Was there ever a time when she didn't want to listen to what I had to say?

The only way I could deal with reality was by hiding from it. I'm not sure if that even counted as "dealing with it," but it's all I had. Every night after work, I'd hang out in my room instead of sitting with her. I thought that if I could avoid talking to her, then I would never get bad news again.

What I didn't consider, however, was that Dad could deliver bad news, too.

It had been an extremely stressful afternoon in my after-school science classroom. On most days, I absolutely loved it, although it wasn't a real, full-time teaching job. Nonetheless, I thought of it as my foot in the door to a real teaching job. But this day was the kind of day when I wondered why the hell I wanted to be a teacher to begin with. My class of first graders was completely off-the-wall. Nothing I said or did could hold their attention for more than three seconds. To make matters worse, this was the day that my boss decided to randomly walk in and observe me. She couldn't have picked a worse time to come into my room. I had a kid falling off his stool and on the verge of breaking his arm, a girl crying in the corner because someone called her "mean," a kid writing on another kid's face with a marker, and one boy trying to climb over the table. My boss was obviously not impressed. The feeling of having no control over your classroom leaves you feeling like you're a terrible teacher.

I couldn't wait for the afternoon to end. The two hours that I worked after school had felt like an entire day. But eventually the day did end, and finally, I was home. I was hungry, exhausted, cranky, and angry all at the same time. I pulled out a pre-made salad from the refrigerator.

Dad must have heard me walk in because he emerged from his man-cave and made his way to the kitchen. I was *so* not in the mood to chat. I pushed past him, a little rudely, to get my salad dressing. He either didn't notice or didn't mind.

Instead, he offered a quick, "Hi."

"Hi," I responded, with no effort to continue the conversation. I poured my salad dressing on, being careful to avoid eye contact with him, and chewed. Took another bite. Chewed.

"She fell again," Dad abruptly informed me. I froze. There was lettuce in my mouth, but it suddenly felt like cement.

I never really knew what he expected me to say to information like this. He told me quite frequently about her falls, but it never got easier to hear. During the one second that my brain was processing the information, I was overwhelmed with emotions, ranging from extreme sadness to furious anger to pure helplessness. How was a twenty-two-year-old supposed to form all of those emotions into a respectful response to her poor father, who had vowed to care for her mother in sickness and in health?

So obviously, I didn't respond. I just let him keep talking. At least I managed to swallow the food in my mouth.

"She can't stand at all anymore," he continued.

I knew that when Dad said she couldn't stand, he didn't mean she couldn't stand on her own. That ability had already been gone for a long time at this point. He meant that she could no longer keep her legs straight enough for us to hold her up. It was kind of like trying to stand a piece of cooked spaghetti upright. You might be able to hold it upright, but once you let go of it, it falls. Mom's legs were just like spaghetti. We needed her to be able to keep them straight so we could move her, adjust her pants, or stretch her legs out. Dad was telling me that her knees were now crippling, which meant she couldn't even lean on him so he could pull her pants up after she'd finished on the toilet.

Finally, my brain reacted. *What the fuck?*

I needed a better reaction. *THINK HARDER, Michelle!*

My next thought was, *Is this for real?* It wasn't much better, but at least it wasn't the F-bomb.

A few seconds went by, and I still hadn't spoken, but again Dad continued. "I don't know what I'm going to do, Michelle." The words seemed to stretch thinly across the space between us and land softly on the floor. I should have bent down picked them up; I should have tried to put the broken pieces back together for him. His gaze was cast downward, his hands rested gently by his sides. He sounded so vulnerable, confused, and broken that all of a sudden, not only did it feel like I'd lost Mom, but like I'd lost Dad, too.

If you ask any little girl who the stronger parent is, Mommy or Daddy, I bet she will respond with "Daddy." Maybe this is because as a kid, "strength" means the size of your arms and your ability to get the pickle jar open. For me, anyway, I always thought of Dad as the stronger parent.

Your dad was the one who never cried no matter what, who you avoided when you did something wrong because you knew he would be harsher with the consequence. He was the brick wall that the whole family leaned on . . . he was the only one strong enough to hold all the weight. He was the one person in a little girl's life who could fix everything that broke. He fixed my Easy-Bake Oven when the light bulb went out and stopped cooking the cookies when I was seven. He fixed my bike when I was ten and needed more air in my tires. He fixed my car before I went to college, and he fixed my hair straightener when I moved back home.

I was twenty-two years old, but I still thought of Dad as the brick wall that I depended on to survive. He was still the one who was supposed to fix everything that went wrong in my life. And yet, no matter how hard he tried, he couldn't fix Mom. None of us could.

I just let his words lay there on the floor, unable to pick them up and try to put them back together. I had no words, no solution, nothing I could do to make any of this better.

How could he pick her up off the toilet and pull her pants up if her legs stayed bent? Why did he have to pick his wife up off the toilet, anyway? Why did his wife get MS? Why did she keep getting worse? When would the horror stop? When would the villain leave Mom alone?

I knew the answer, or at least . . . I thought I did. It was flashing in my head like a bright red neon sign.

Dad would be able to stop taking care of her, and she would finally stop getting worse when the villain had completely taken her down. Until that time, the villain would continue to do everything possible to suck the person out of Mom. It would keep trying until there was nothing left of Mom but the empty shell of a human being, at which point, the villain would have created its masterpiece, and it would leave Mom to die.

I was sure of it. If someone asked me to bet a million dollars on it, I would have. I thought MS would win when it tried to kill her.

But I was wrong.

May 2, 2013
Dear Michelle,

I've had this book for way too long without writing. You've graduated from college! You have been teaching science at the after-school program in Nashua. So it's time for you to reflect on what is reality now. Hopes and dreams of college still exist. But now the real world has entered into the perfect utopia created by campus life.

I hope you are finding your way. I hope you are discovering the possibilities and realizing where you fit. Your relationship with Tyler is growing and changing, too. You both seem to share the same dreams and goals. And you have similar moral compasses that guide you. You know that I just want you to be happy.

Everything in life does not have to be a struggle. Just keep things manageable. It's when things get too big, and you feel like you're out of control that you'll become unhappy. That's not to say don't think BIG and dream BIG! You can do BIG things! You deserve the best! But in reality, you'll be the happiest if you keep life simple.

I really do not want this to be about me. But every day I think about how MS affects you. I wonder, if I was well, would we do more together? Or is it because I'm sick that we do what we do? I don't want to cramp your style. I don't want to think about all the things we may have done together.

Perhaps, if I were well, we would both be too busy to be together. Perhaps this crazy MS shit has forced us to slow down and appreciate things. I know I have been reclusive and I worry about the example I set for you and Alex. It's taking me so long to figure out how to live a life that is not really living.

I'm not dead. I still feel joy and pride watching all my kids. But I feel like a fly on the wall. Watching things go on around me, but knowing I can't jump in and join the party. Again, maybe that's a good thing—who needs a crazy old mother hanging around?!

Anyway, we are both navigating the crazy MS journey. Sucks to be you! Lol! Not!

I hope you dance!
I love you!
Mom

CHAPTER TWENTY-FOUR
MICHELLE

Living at home after college wasn't completely terrible. I loved the fact that I could save money. Dad cooked me dinner quite frequently (although it was almost *always* chicken). It was where my dog lived. Alex was there with me until he was twenty-seven and bought his own place, and I liked hanging out with him. I didn't have a curfew or particularly strict rules to obey. My parents just asked that I showed them respect. I did, and they respected me in return.

Dad and I's relationship had evolved significantly ever since the villain had come into our lives. When I thought about what Dad was like when I was a kid, a mixture of pleasant and not-so-pleasant memories flooded back to me. He was incredible at drawing illustrations, a skill that I definitely did not inherit. I remembered asking him for help with all my school projects that required illustrations of any kind. One report, in fourth grade, was about a made-up animal that had varying evolutionary traits. A fish with paws! A shark with legs! Of course, I wanted my animal to fly. I combined a pelican and a pig to form a "pelipig," and then asked Dad to draw it. It was an odd, pink creature with a pig's body and pelican wings. It was something I had conjured in my own imagination, and I wasn't sure if he would be able to draw what I was seeing in my head. But Dad managed to draw it perfectly.

I remembered watching *Cops* with Dad and Alex while Mom worked retail at night. I was only in first grade, but Dad didn't see any problems with having me watch "bad guys" get tased, beaten and arrested because it was "what they had comin' to them." He thought it would teach me how to *not be*. He also let me watch *The Simpsons* and *Seinfeld*, even though they were totally not age-appropriate. But he was a good dad, and he loved me. He told me he was proud of me every chance he got. He told me I was beautiful and always believed in me. There was no doubt in my mind that he loved me as much as he could.

For a long time, he had a horrible temper, and his mood could flip on a dime. His patience was thin, and his tolerance for ignorance was even thinner. I remember him yelling . . . a lot. Yelling at me. Yelling at my friends. Yelling at Alex, Mom, the dog, the telemarketer who dared to call him at exactly the wrong moment. I could recall many times growing up when I had friends over to play, and Dad would start yelling about something right in front of them. The topics that caused him to become angry him were stupid and insignificant, like something wasn't put away correctly, or my shoes were blocking his ability to walk through the door. Little stuff.

When I was young, I was afraid his yelling might mean he would break something or hurt someone. He never did hurt anyone, and he only broke the occasional glass dish, always by accident. But his voice was loud and, as a little girl, it was the scariest thing I had ever known. Sometimes I would yell back, but eventually, I learned that fighting with him was an impossible waste of energy and that it would never make him stop yelling.

I'd try to explain to my friends who were around when he was yelling that he didn't mean anything by it and that it would blow over quickly. Most of them understood. As I grew older, I realized that his yelling was more of a coping mechanism for him to deal with the stress and struggles that daily life presented. Knowing this, I started not being able to take it seriously. When he came home from work and started yelling, I'd just walk away and wait for him to calm himself down. The older I got, the stupider his yelling became. It started being humorous to me that he could get so worked up about the smallest things. I learned to laugh, shake my head, and wait for the fog in his head to clear.

I became used to the sound of him yelling. What I couldn't get used to, no matter how hard I tried, was the sound of Mom yelling. Because when she yelled, it wasn't out of anger or frustration, as it was with Dad. It was a completely different kind of scream.

One afternoon, I was in the kitchen eating lunch and getting ready to go to work at the after-school program. Dad was in the basement doing some work for his company which he had started running from home so he could take care of Mom. Mom was in her bathroom when the silence in the kitchen, on the opposite side of the house, was abruptly interrupted.

It sounded like the honking from a train that was passing by right in front of you . . . loud enough to make me want to cover your ears, scary enough to make me want to run away.

Mom was screaming at the top of her lungs, repetitively, without stopping. "HELLLLLLLLP!" I heard her cry. My body responded immediately to her first scream, but she kept screaming. "HELLLLLLLP!" "HELLLLLLLLLLLLLLLLLLLP!"

I'm coming! I thought to myself. Her yell started sounding like the train was moving at full-speed. It was coming off its track. The train conductor had lost control, and no one on board could gain it back. The train shook the entire house and made the hair on the back of my neck stand up.

STOP SCREAMING! I wanted to yell back at her.

It was like when you were a kid, and the train was passing by. At first, you made the motion for the train conductor to sound the horn. You were okay the first time he did it, but after that, it just sounded loud, and you wished he would stop. Once was enough—no need to continue on a million times.

"HELLLLLLLLLLLLLLP!" The conductor honked again.

I would never get used to the shrill sound of Mom screaming for help. It was like nails on a chalkboard, except not only did my ears feel like they were bleeding, but my heart as well. Her voice was dry and crackly. There was something different about this cry. It was too urgent . . . too scary. I had never heard her scream like this before.

I threw down the piece of bread that I had been nibbling on. I aimed for my plate and missed it. It landed on the floor. I left it there and jumped off my barstool. I broke into a sprint toward her bedroom. The hallway from the kitchen to her bedroom was long, but I covered it in about five strides. I reached her room and heard Dad rushing upstairs from the basement, skipping steps to get there as fast as he could, too.

How's Your Mom?

I reached her first. She was sitting on the toilet, naked, crying. She must have just showered, which meant her energy was in low supply. It looked like she had fallen over to her right side, but she caught herself. She was holding onto one of the railings that Dad had installed to the sides of the toilet. She was grasping the railing as tight as she could, but it was clear that she had no strength, and in another few seconds, had Dad or I not been here, she would have fallen on her side and probably broken her arm.

At first, I didn't know where I should touch her. She was naked all over, and I felt extremely awkward. I managed to grab her by her sides and pull her up onto the toilet. Just as I returned her to safety, Dad rushed in to pick up the pieces. Mom started crying hysterically while trying to explain to me that she simply leaned too far over and lost her balance. I was too upset to listen, so I slowly backed away and left Dad to listen to her sobs. I heard him say, "It's okay, baby," and unbeknownst to them, right there at that moment, they made me believe in love.

I broke down in the hallway—half-listening to Mom's sobs, half-wishing I couldn't hear them. My knees gave out, and I couldn't make it any further. I collapsed. I cried on the hardwood floors . . . the silent kind that you could almost convince yourself wasn't really happening. I kept crying until I heard Dad start to walk out of the bathroom. No one could see me like that—I needed to move.

I managed to stand and walk back toward the kitchen. Dad didn't see me and went right back downstairs, probably to have the same reaction. He wouldn't let his little girl see him cry either. We pretended we were fooling each other. We were both too strong to cry.

About an hour later, Mom emerged in the kitchen for lunch. I was putting on my jacket and getting ready to head out the door. She explained that a loss of strength and energy often happened when she did her exercises (as recommended by her physical therapist), especially on a day when she showered. If she didn't move her body, she would lose the ability. Yet stretching and moving took so much out of her that it was really a lose-lose situation.

"I'm sorry," she said softly. "Thanks for coming to help me so quickly."

She shouldn't have felt the need to thank me or apologize. Did she not see how proud of her I was every single day for continuing to live the way she did?

"It's okay," I said. It seemed weird to say *you're welcome* for a decision I'd made when I had no choice.

"Thanks, Shell," Dad said as he entered the kitchen. "You're a big help."

He shouldn't have had to thank me either. He was the one who picked up all the broken pieces all the rest of the time when I wasn't around, but he didn't seem to mind.

I gave him a nod without saying anything. He began whistling and preparing himself a tuna sandwich for lunch. He was acting as if everything was completely fine . . . as if a train hadn't just crashed into our whole house.

I watched him, remaining silent, wondering how he could possibly appear to be in such a good mood already. I was still in a million pieces and completely shaken up. I felt so broken inside that I was seriously contemplating if "My mom almost fell" was a legitimate excuse to call out of work. I decided that if Dad was fine, then I was, too.

I pulled on my boots. "Hope you have a good day at school! Don't worry, I'll take care of Mom. It will take more than that to bring me down!" he practically sang out to me while he bit into his tuna sandwich.

At that moment, I wished he could take those words back. Because before the words even hit the air, I thought, *be careful what you wish for.*

How's Your Mom?

TAMMY

It was like there was a little person inside of me screaming out, "I am here! I am here! I am here!" like in the book *Horton Hears a Who*. I am a Who living in Whoville. I think. I talk. I read. I watch. I listen.

When I try to do anything, my body fails me.

But *I am here.*

CHAPTER TWENTY-FIVE
MICHELLE

On the days where she was really well-rested, she would feel great. She would question whether or not she was actually sick. On the good days, I could take her out of the house all by myself.

One hot summer day, while I was still living at my parents' house, Dad let me take Mom to get some routine blood work done. Since Mom had been getting a dose of chemotherapy every month, the doctors required that she get blood work done once a week to make sure everything was okay. I loved being able to help Dad with stuff like this. He would have normally brought her to this type of appointment, but I let him have the day off. Taking care of Mom was practically a full-time job. He was thrilled to go to a classic car show instead.

The first step was getting Mom out of the house. It doesn't seem like it would be a complicated thing, but it was honestly more work than eighty-five percent of my workouts at the gym.

It was hot, and Mom didn't do well in the heat. I knew that if I didn't take precautions, by the end of the day, she would have melted into a pool of deadweight, and I would be in charge of making sure she didn't fall down.

It was nine a.m., and Dad had gotten her all showered and dressed for me. I met her in the kitchen and thought, *bring it on.*

First and foremost, we needed to put her shoes on—no easy task. She'd invested in a pair of canvas Tom's . . . not because they donated a pair to a child in need whenever someone buys a pair, but because they were stretchy and fit her swollen purple feet. They also didn't have any laces or Velcro, which was a necessity because her fingers didn't work so she couldn't tie her own shoes or even strap-on Velcro.

After a short struggle, her shoes were safe and secure. She looked up at me and waited for me to pick her up.

I bent down, wrapped my arms around her and lifted her out of her electric wheelchair. We couldn't bring the electric wheelchair outside, so we had a normal wheelchair that we took out instead. I'd already set this chair up behind me. As Mom clung to my neck, I could feel her body pressing up against me for support. I needed to lean her torso onto mine, assuming responsibility for all her body weight, as if she had no legs at all. Then, I used her bending legs to hop her one-hundred-eighty degrees around, and carefully dropped her into the other wheelchair. If she weighed too much, I wouldn't have been able to do it. Fortunately, she only weighed about a hundred pounds. Her size-four pants were falling down as I began to place her in the chair. I made a mental note to buy her some new pants since she was now clearly a size two or maybe even a zero.

Once we were in the "outside wheelchair," as I called it, it was time to leave the house. Dad had installed a ramp that covered the three stairs leading from our kitchen into the garage. It was short and extremely steep. This was the first time I'd rolled the wheelchair down the ramp, and I was terrified that I wouldn't be able to do it. Dad's shiny, bright red 1970 Chevelle SS was parked in the garage just feet from the end of the ramp, and if I lost control of the wheelchair, I might have fallen back into the car and made some sort of mark or fingerprint on it. That couldn't happen because Dad would *actually* kill me.

I took a deep breath, walked halfway down the ramp, and got into a lunge position so most of the weight from the chair would be on my legs. I held the handles of the chair and guided it quickly down the ramp. Thankfully, I didn't hit the car. I was beyond excited but forced myself to keep my chill and continue moving.

Once we were in the garage, the heat hit me like a ton of bricks, and I suddenly remembered that I couldn't have Mom melting before I got her in the car. I let go of the wheelchair and sprinted to turn on the air conditioner on. I really should have done that ten minutes before, but better late than never, right? I wheeled her over to the passenger side door, positioned the chair just right, put the brakes on and bent down to her level.

"Wrap your arms around my neck. Hold onto me," I told

her firmly.

She did as I requested, and I lifted her straight up, did the hop-dance to get her turned around again, and placed her in the car. Her feet were still dangling outside, so I picked them up and turn her body, so she was facing forward. As I closed her door, I silently congratulated myself for not dropping her.

With Mom sitting safely in the Mazda, I needed to fit the wheelchair into my car. It was supposed to fold up pretty easily, and the foot holders were supposed to come off to make it easier for the chair to fit in my back seat. Dad had told me they were easy to take off, but he hadn't shown me how to do it. As I struggled with it, I thought about how Mom was probably roasting in the car while I couldn't figure out how to make the chair fit into the door.

It took me a while to figure out the foot holders. I tried simply popping them off, but I couldn't figure out how. Then I thought something was supposed to fold and tried pressing in odd places. Nothing seemed to fold. I noticed a shiny silver handle and tried pulling it. I had no luck. Maybe I was supposed to push it? That didn't work. My mind raced. *What was I doing wrong?*

I pulled. Pushed. Twisted. Turned. Pinched my finger. My frustration grew, and I worried about Mom. I thought she must have been hot, and she was probably wondering what was taking me so long. After about two minutes, it became straight-up embarrassing that the foot holders were still on the chair and the chair was still not in the car.

After another full minute went by, I figured out how to get the foot holders off. I realized how easy it should have been and felt a surge of self-hatred rush through me.

Hastily, I folded the chair. I needed to lift it up and put it in the backseat. At that moment, I really wished I were stronger. No, I wished I had bigger biceps. *That would be cool.* I had a sudden vision of myself at the gym, lifting weights that were heavier than ten pounds. I could be one of the girls who weren't afraid of the free-weight area, and people would call me the Girl with the Toned Arms. The best part of being the Girl with the Toned Arms would be that lifting Mom would be so much easier. Yes. I definitely need-

How's Your Mom?

ed to go to the gym more. I would start tomorrow, I told myself.

Suddenly it dawned on me that another thirty seconds had gone by and I still hadn't put the stupid wheelchair in the car. It felt so heavy, and my arms were starting to ache. It wouldn't fit in the backseat where I was trying to shove it. I couldn't get it to lie down flat correctly. I needed to turn it ninety degrees. As soon as I turned it, dirt rained down from the wheels and landed all over the seat. So vacuuming my car yesterday in an effort to impress Mom had definitely been worth it.

For a moment, I considered asking for help. Surely she could have turned around and told me how to position the chair because she'd seen Dad do it a million times.

As I opened my mouth to speak, my eyes registered her face. Her eyes were closed, and she was slouched way down in her seat. I realized that she couldn't help me. Even if she wanted to turn around to look at the situation, I didn't think she could have without my help. It was just another thing I'd have to figure out on my own.

I kept twisting the chair until finally, after a long struggle, I managed to fit it on the seat and slam the door shut. Another surge of pride ran through me, and I forced myself to move along.

Growing up, car rides were my favorite time because Mom and I didn't have to look at each other. I could say whatever I wanted without worrying about what her face looked like when I told her things. I'd tell her all about my friends and fill her in on all the latest drama of my life—the good and bad decisions I had made lately. She listened and always said the right thing.

But on this particular day, she kept her eyes closed and remained silent, obviously fighting the nausea caused by the heat from the sun shining through the window on her side of the car. I wanted to say something, I wanted to talk to her, but I didn't want to make her feel any sicker than she probably already did. So I just drove and tried to ignore the stab in my chest when I looked at her, so tiny and tired in the seat beside me.

We finally made it to the parking lot where the lab was located. I pulled in the parking lot and located the wheelchair ramp from the pavement to the sidewalk. I parked next to it and realized it was about a mile away from the entrance of the lab. *Awesome,* I thought. Whoever designed the exterior of the plaza did a fantastic job. Seriously, this was my workout for the day.

I left the air conditioner running for Mom while I struggled to get the chair out of the car. I had to put those stupid foot holders on again. Taking them off had been hard. But putting them back on was SO MUCH HARDER. It should have been simple, but I could never get them turned the right way. I'd never been good at geometry, and I could never figure out which way they should face. Every time I did it, I was reminded of the game Tetris, where the puzzle pieces were falling, and you had to turn them quickly enough and form them in a perfect row so they lay flat on the bottom, and the screen didn't fill up. I sucked at it. I blamed my lack of geometry skills for the thirty seconds it took me to put the foot holders on.

Again, I told Mom to put her arms around my neck, and I placed her in the chair. I rolled her to the door of the lab and noticed a sketchy-looking guy standing next to us outside the door. I caught his eye and wondered if he would open the door. Instead, he stared at us. At me, maybe. My shorts *were* kind of short.

I scoffed just loudly enough for him to hear it and sense my disapproval, and shot him a dirty look for good measure. I wondered what was going on inside his head, if anything at all. He was either confused that such a young girl was pushing her mom in a wheelchair, and so taken aback that all he could do was freeze, or he was checking me out. Either way, I was not impressed. I wanted to say, "Hey idiot, can you open the damn door?" but instead I struggled to open it myself.

We were already in the building when he finally jerked into motion and took hold of the door. He was really about five seconds too late, but I said thanks anyway.

People. Honestly.

I found Mom's name on the sign-in sheet. I had to forge her signature since the clipboard was chained to the counter and couldn't reach her lap. I wondered if someone would seriously steal a clipboard.

When it was our turn, the phlebotomist approached us and told me to bring Mom to the first door on the left. As I pushed her, one of those awkward silences crept up the hallway between us. I could sense that small talk was on the way. Just as the phlebotomist was about to ask us how we were doing and what the weather outside was like, I accidentally crashed Mom's foot into the side of the door frame. The phlebotomist made a joke about me being a bad driver. *Ha, ha. Never heard that one before!* I thought. Whatever . . . at least we'd escaped the small talk.

Casually, the phlebotomist stuck a needle in Mom's arm. Mom said she didn't feel a thing. As I watched her, cool, calm and collected demeanor, I thought about how she really was my hero. Just the thought of having a needle stabbed into me made me want to cry, and usually, I passed out every time I got a shot. But Mom didn't hyperventilate, cry hysterically, or need the nurse to awkwardly hand her tissues and a juice box like I usually did, so she was done with her blood work in about twenty seconds. *Must be nice,* I thought to myself, and for the first time in years, I found myself feeling jealous of Mom.

I began wheeling her out and slammed her foot into the door frame again. The phlebotomist made another joke about me needing driving lessons. I laughed the fakest laugh that's ever been laughed while wishing she would shut up.

Before I knew it, we were back at the door. I looked at it for a moment, realizing a door that opens inward is a bit trickier to tackle by yourself, and wondered if anyone who was sitting in the lobby two feet away would stand up and hold it for me. No one did, but it was fine. I managed to get Mom back to the car, struggled with the foot holders again, put the chair in the car, and drove her home.

As we pulled into the driveway, she sang out loud, "Home again, home again, jiggity jig!" *That damn phrase,* I thought as I ignored her completely, too agitated to even acknowledge it.

By that point, she was a soggy log. It wasn't easy to lift her out of the car, hold her up, and straighten her legs at the same time, then do the hop-dance to turn her around and put her in the wheelchair again. But somehow, I managed fine.

Before she knew it, I had pushed her up the ramp, parked her at her big, comfy chair in the living room, lifted her up from the wheelchair and plopped her down in the living room chair. I picked her feet up first, pushed the footrest closer toward her and brought her some iced tea. "Thanks," she offered softly.

Immediately, she closed her eyes. She began to fall asleep while I was still standing right in front of her. This had been a big day for her. It had been a big day for me, too.

How's Your Mom?

CHAPTER TWENTY-SIX

TAMMY

I liked being in Tammy World best.

I had been in many places, but I had never been in cahoots. Apparently, you can't go alone. You have to be in cahoots with someone else. I couldn't keep a secret or a straight face so everyone could see right through any charade I may have been attempting.

I'd also never been incognito. I heard no one recognizes you there. I did enjoy having fun, and that generally requires some degree of exposure.

I had, however, been insane. They didn't have an airport; you had to be driven there. I made several trips there, thanks to my friends, family, and work.

I would have like to go to conclusions, but you had to jump, and I wasn't too much on physical activity anymore.

I had also been in doubt. That was a sad place to go, and I tried not to visit there too often.

I had been inflexible, but only when it was very important to stand firm.

Sometimes I was incapable, and I went there more often as I grew older.

One of my favorite places to be was in suspense. It really got the adrenaline flowing and pumped up the old heart. At my age, I needed all the stimuli I could get.

I may have been incontinent, but I was just passing through and, fortunately, I did not stay in that place very long.

Some may say I was in denial, but that place was easily confused with being in survivor mode. The riptide of MS taught me to relax, rather than fight. The progression advanced on its own agenda.

So I was okay with being here in Tammy World. It was safe and comfy there.

CHAPTER TWENTY-SEVEN
MICHELLE

"Hi, Michelle," Mom called out to me from her chair in the living room.

"Hi, Mom," I mumbled back. I had just walked in the door, my hands were full of stuff, my key was stuck in the lock, and my dumb dog was blocking the entryway trying to say hello, making it impossible for me to walk inside.

I had left the after-school program and was working as an assistant teacher in a third-grade classroom. It was the most perfect school I could ever dream of, and for the first time in my life, I truly loved my job. But today, I didn't get home until five, and I was completely exhausted. It had been one of those days when no matter how many cups of coffee I drank, I felt like I could never wake up. I would walk into a room and forget what I was doing. I'd put down my coffee, walk away from it, and have no idea where I left it. I'd walk around a corner without paying attention and smack right into someone. AGAIN AND AGAIN. It was blonde moment after blonde moment. It was an entire blonde day.

"MOVE, Honeybee!" I yelled out to my dog, who was still standing in my way. I gave her a light nudge and pushed past her. I dropped my bags down on the chair and began to take off my jacket.

"How was your day?" Mom asked quietly from the living room.

Without even stopping to think, I responded with an automatic "good," and mentally declared our conversation over. I headed toward the refrigerator, opened it, and grabbed a pre-made salad.

I didn't want to talk to her. Talking to her only reminded me that I wasn't talking to *her*, but what was left of her. She wasn't the mom she used to be. Talking to her only reminded me of that.

Apart from acting like a huge bitch, I was also scared. I wasn't as brave as I wanted everyone to think I was. Truthfully, I was afraid I'd never understand how something could take away everything you are and have. I didn't *want* to understand it, either.

I'd always believed that you are the sum of your experiences. So when your experiences diminish, and all you're left with are empty days, sitting in a chair playing on your iPad, is that what you become? Are you the sum of your empty days? When I talked to Mom, that's what she seemed like. She was no longer the voice of reason and wisdom. Her voice only echoed the emptiness of her days. The same voice that once soothed my worries and comforted me made me want to run away in a fury of anger. It frustrated me endlessly. But I couldn't always run away from it. Some days I had to stand there and endure her meaningless words and pretend what she was saying made any sense. Usually, it didn't make much sense, not to me anyway. Maybe it was because I wasn't being patient enough . . . if I could just relax and try to listen a little harder, I would have been able to hear what she was trying to say, to fill the void that she struggled to overcome.

But sometimes it was too hard and I couldn't. I couldn't always be so patient because all I was ever thinking about was *why the hell she can't speak normally in the first place?* It was so unfair and downright cruel for someone to have to endure that kind of frustration. Truthfully, it was crueler to her than to me, because she was as conscious of her shortcomings as I was. She knew how I used to look to her for advice, and realized the lack of communication between us had dwindled because of her inability to speak to me. She knew it was her fault, and yet there was nothing she could do to make it better. She was stuck. I was stuck. We were both stuck in the exact same place, but it felt like we were miles apart.

CHAPTER TWENTY-EIGHT

CHRIS

By 2015, my wife's condition had gotten pretty bad. We weren't denying it or hiding it from anyone anymore. She was completely wheelchair-bound and only had use of her right hand. I had to lift her to get her anywhere: the toilet, shower, you name it. She didn't go out much because it was too hard. It took too much out of her. Plus, since our kids had both moved out and purchased their own homes, I was the only person taking care of her. Fortunately, Alex moved only a few miles down the road, and Michelle was only a half-hour away, so they still came over frequently. If one of the kids was there, they could watch her. Still, she *let me* go to my car shows, even if the kids weren't there. I'd only go for a few hours, but I never left her alone unless she was safely in bed. It's the only place I trusted her not to get hurt.

Every now and then, there would be a car show on a weekend. It would start around eleven, and I'd be home by two. In August, my favorite car show was going to fall on the same day that Tammy's dad would be having his ninety-second birthday party. Michelle would be able to come over, get Tammy ready for the party, and drive her down to Massachusetts while I was at my show. It was all planned out. Michelle would take good care of her; she told me I didn't have to worry. But I *always* worried.

After I left, Michelle decided to go out for half an hour, and she left Tammy in her wheelchair. I never left Tammy in her wheelchair. When Tammy was in her wheelchair, she could get herself into trouble. But Michelle didn't quite understand that.

Later, I couldn't help but wonder what our futures would have been like if only Michelle hadn't left Tammy in her wheelchair that day.

PART THREE
CLOSING THE SALE
AUGUST 2015–DECEMBER 2015

CHAPTER TWENTY-NINE

MICHELLE

It was a sunny Sunday morning, warm and breezy with zero humidity in the air. It was my favorite kind of Sunday. I had told Mom I would take her to my grandfather's ninety-second birthday party. We had a very clear plan. I was to arrive at my parents' house at ten, help Mom finished getting dressed, and then drive her to the party. Dad was going to head to a car show. I didn't mind if he left us alone. I was happy to help. I was so glad he had a hobby. More importantly, I was glad he had an escape from his reality.

"Hi, Dad," I called as I walked into my house, which hadn't really been *my house* for a year and a half. I had moved out the previous June. But it would always be my home.

"Shell!" he exclaimed with open arms. He always greeted me with a hug and a smile. Even if it had only been a week since my last visit, Dad was always so happy to see me. It was something I knew I'd never forget.

We made casual small talk as I gave Honeybee a good pat. Her tiny stump moved up and down as she leaned against my legs. She was part boxer, and whoever had owned her before we did had cut off her tail. All she had left was a tiny stump.

I found Mom sitting in her wheelchair, working on a digital scrapbook page on her iPad. I walked to her and gave her a hug, feeling genuinely happy to see her. To my surprise and delight, she was actually already dressed. Though I was relieved that Dad checked a chore off of my list, I was also a little angry that I had busted my butt to get out of the door when I really didn't need to be here until later. Now I would have an hour to kill before it was time to leave for my grandfather's, whom I called Zaydie.

Almost immediately after I arrived, Dad was out the door. He couldn't wait to get to this car show; it was one of his favorites. He said good-bye to Mom and me, and we watched his car roll slowly down the street. The roar of his engine was so loud we could hear it from a mile away.

Mom seemed like she was in a good mood. She had a lot of energy, or so it appeared, and she really was pretty much ready to go. I thought it would be a great idea if we had coffee for our road trip, and since we had extra time, I thought I should go pick some up.

"Mom, can I go get us Starbucks?"

"Oh . . . okay. Sure." She hesitated, and I wasn't sure why.

"You're all ready, right? We have extra time?" I asked, trying to figure out why she was so hesitant for me to leave.

"Yeah, I'm just about ready."

"Okay, cool. I'll be back in twenty minutes. Will you be all right?"

"Oh, yeah, I'll be fine," she assured me.

As I closed the door behind me, the only thing on my mind was coffee.

The Starbucks drive-thru line was insanely long. It wrapped around the entire parking lot. I figured, since I had time to kill, that wait would be no big deal. I listened to the radio and tried to ignore the minutes that were ticking by. I hoped Mom was all right.

After ten minutes, it was finally my turn to place my order. Once I did, there was really no turning back. I ordered two small iced coffees with skim milk only. Another ten minutes passed before I reached the window. With two coffees in my cup holders, I finally headed back home. The trip had taken thirty minutes, even though the Starbucks was only two miles away.

With a coffee in each hand, I had a hard time getting the front door unlocked. I dropped my keychain twice before finally fitting it correctly in the lock. As I stepped inside, Honeybee blocked my way as she always did.

I took a few steps to the counter and put the coffees and my keys down. Mom wasn't in the kitchen anymore.

"Mom?" I called out. I didn't hear an answer.

"Mom?" I asked, growing more anxious with every passing second. I walked toward her bedroom, where I saw her wheelchair parked next to her dresser, her sock drawer pulled open. She was lying in a crumpled heap on the floor. She must have fallen forward out of her wheelchair. She was crying.

"Oh my G-d, Mom!" I called. "Are you okay?"

"I can't move," she sputtered. She was hysterical. Her weight seemed to be centered entirely on her left shoulder. I could tell she was in pain, but I had no idea how much.

Before I could get to her, I needed to back her wheelchair away. Some of her weight had been kept in place by its position, so once I moved it, she fell slightly more forward, and she wailed in agony.

"I'm sorry! I need to get behind you!" I tried to explain.

Once I had enough room to squeeze behind her and the dresser, I reached my arms through her hers and attempted to lift her torso up.

"OW!" she screamed, and I froze.

"What?" I asked, stupidly.

She couldn't speak. There were only tears. I realized something must have happened to her shoulder.

Instead of trying to get my arms in her underarms, I left her arms at her sides and wrapped mine around her entire body. I could tell this still hurt her, but at least I managed to get her to a sitting position. I had to lean her back against my hand for support so she wouldn't fall backwards.

I had no idea how I was going to pick her up. I stood over her and experimented with a few different positions before my mind started racing.

"Mom, I don't know how I'm going to pick you up," I finally admitted.

For a moment, she was able to stop crying. She looked up at me with sad, bloodshot eyes, and for the first time in my life, I realized how truly helpless she must have felt.

I could have called someone. I could have run to my neighbors' house. But I didn't want to. My stubborn independence struck again. I took a moment to pause and formulate a plan. Feeling slightly inspired, I pulled her body toward the side of the bed and leaned her back up against it. I sat on the edge of the bed with her body between my legs and pulled her up to the bed. Still straddling her, I pulled her wheelchair closer to us and successfully transitioned her to it.

She was safe, or so I thought. I examined her shoulder and didn't see anything wrong with it. As time passed, she stopped crying and seemed to recover. She explained that she had been trying to put her socks on. She leaned forward, and . . . well, I knew the rest. All she was trying to do was put her socks on.

Soon after, Alex and his cross-my-fingers-future-sister-in-law, Christine, came over. We were going to drive down to the party together. We told them what had happened, but we thought we could still go to the birthday party. Alex helped me get her outside and, together, we tried to lift her into his car. She screamed in agony. We couldn't go.

Instead, we settled her in the living room with an ice pack on her shoulder. She told us she thought she pulled a muscle. She told us she would be fine.

But she wasn't.

For the next two months, she awoke in the middle of the night in pain. Her shoulder had frequent spasms that caused her to scream out in discomfort. We tried to get her to go to the doctor. She didn't want to. Maybe she was afraid of trying to get into the car again.

Months passed. We celebrated her fifty-fourth birthday, and Dad wondered what to do. She was in pain all the time. Christine, a PA student specializing in orthopedics, warned Mom that it looked like she had a dislocated shoulder. It didn't matter. We couldn't get her to go to the hospital.

Until one Friday night, when we had to go to the emergency room.

CHAPTER THIRTY

CHRIS

I had had enough of this bullshit. She hadn't slept through the night in months, and I couldn't stand to see her in so much pain. It was like a switch flipped inside of me, and I thought, *this has to end.*

So I brought her to our family's doctor office, and they immediately told me to put her in the front seat of my car and bring her to the hospital. They told me that an orthopedic surgeon, Dr. Tim, would be standing there waiting for me.

"Why?" I asked.

"Because her shoulder is separated." As if it were obvious. *You idiot, her shoulder is separated. Of course it fucking is.*

I loaded her into the car and drove her to the emergency room at the hospital. The doctor couldn't operate that night because they needed special tools to complete an operation to reset her shoulder. They assembled their team and made a plan to operate on her shoulder the next day.

I pulled out my phone and texted my kids. My text simply said "Mom in emergency room. Come if you can."

CHAPTER THIRTY-ONE

MICHELLE

I didn't know what to think when I walked into the emergency room that night. On the one hand, I was relieved that Mom was finally getting her shoulder checked out. On the other, I felt so sorry for her. I hated that I'd been right when we told her something was very wrong.

I couldn't believe how tiny the emergency room was. I hadn't been in one since I was seven years old and fell off Alex's bed. I'd sliced my armpit open on his Ghostbusters house, and Dad had to take me to the emergency room to get stitches. I didn't remember it at all. I was shocked that it wasn't a real room; it was only a nook with a curtain. Dad, Alex, and I could barely fit in there all at once.

Mom was exhausted. The doctors had already done a few x-rays on her by the time I got there. Her doctor was Dr. Tim. He was a nice man. Mom thought he was very handsome. He specialized in orthopedics, and he was the one who explained her x-rays to us. On a piece of black-and-white paper, Mom's shoulder and collarbone were pictured. I couldn't understand what was wrong with the picture, so Dr. Tim pulled out a blue pen and drew on it for me. He outlined her collarbone and told me that it was probably fractured from her fall that day. Amazingly, though, it was healing.

As the collarbone was healing, however, the MS had other plans. It caused Mom to have intense spasms in her shoulder, and Dr. Tim thought the spasms were actually what caused her shoulder joint to come out of her socket. He circled the joint where her shoulder was, and showed me the nook where it should have been settled in. The ball was very visibly not resting inside the socket. *Damn you, MS.*

He wasn't very worried, and as he explained the surgery she would need to have, he sounded very confident. He explained that he would put the ball back in its socket, but since the spasms had caused her ligaments around the socket to stretch out so much, he would need to attach a piece of bone to the socket to keep the ball in place. Otherwise, it would just roll right out again.

He would need to do a bone graft; a standard, relatively easy surgery, or so it seemed to me. As with any surgery, there was a risk of infection, which we immediately dismissed because we knew she *needed* the surgery. So she spent the night in the hospital and was prepped for surgery the following morning.

Surgery: a simple solution to end a chapter of our lives.

Or so we thought.

CHAPTER THIRTY-TWO

CHRIS

The shoulder surgery went well. Tammy was released from the hospital two days later with a new shoulder sling and a repaired shoulder socket. We also received at-home nurses, who came to check on her.

A few days after the surgery, a nurse came to check on her as instructed. She noticed immediately that Tammy had a fever and hadn't produced anything from her kidneys in twenty-four hours. She turned to me and said, "I have to call your wife an ambulance."

What the fuck are you talking about? I thought.

"I think she has an infection," she explained.

So we called an ambulance. We told the nurse not to call 9-1-1 because we didn't want the lights and sirens to alarm the neighbors. Our neighbors still came out and expressed their concerns.

We brought her in, and I texted my kids the news again. They arrived at the emergency room minutes later, and we all waited while the doctors tried to figure out what was wrong. She was in and out of consciousness and in tons of pain.

That night, they admitted her to a room on the fifth floor, and we stayed with her as long as we could. Eventually, the doctors told us to go home and rest. They told us that they had no idea what was wrong.

CHAPTER THIRTY-THREE
MICHELLE

The following morning, Dad, Alex, and I made our separate ways to the hospital to check on Mom. I was worried about her all night, knowing that she wasn't able to eat much of the pudding I'd tried to feed her the night before, and knowing how sick she had felt when I said goodnight to her. Seeing her that sick scared me.

Dad got to the hospital earlier than I did because he always woke up much earlier than me. Shortly after arriving, he texted Alex and me, saying that something was wrong with her brain. He said, "She's had a complete personality change."

A complete personality change? Something wrong with her brain? What did that even mean? How could that happen overnight?

I flew out of bed and got dressed as quickly as I could. I stormed into the hospital, completely ignoring the lady at the front desk, and headed straight to the elevators. I pressed the button marked "five" and waited for the doors to close. The elevator moved much too slowly.

Finally, I reached the fifth floor. As the doors opened and I momentarily struggled to remember which way her room was located, I could suddenly hear her screaming. *Was that my mom?* She sounded like a crazy person. Maybe it wasn't her. As I got closer, I heard the familiar tone of her voice, but still couldn't believe it was her.

"I need someone to pray with me!" she screamed. Her screams echoed down the hallways, and I thought that if I were a patient here, or a child visiting my parent, I would have been scared of her. "I need to say the Mi Shebeirach!" The Mi Shebeirach was the Jewish prayer for the sick. If I had any remaining doubts about whether or not it was her, now I was sure.

I walked in the room, but she didn't even notice. The nurses and hospital staff looked at me, probably wishing I knew what to do. Instead of greeting me like a normal person, Mom screamed at the air surrounding me.

"Hi, Mom," I cautiously ventured.

"GET A RABBI!" she yelled. "ALL I NEED IS A RABBI!"

The air around her felt cold and fierce. I was afraid to get too close to her. The sound of her yelling completely terrified me. I took a tiny step closer to her, noticing that she couldn't seem to look right at me. "Mom? What's going on?"

"MICHELLE, GET A RABBI!" she shouted, still not able to look me in the eye. And yet, she knew I was there. Or did she?

I looked over my left and right shoulders, hoping a rabbi would magically appear. I even walked into the hallway and looked around. *What was I looking for? A rabbi vending machine?*

"Mom, there aren't any rabbis," I explained, coming back. "I looked in the hallway," I added for good measure.

I wished I knew the prayer well enough myself, but I didn't. I hadn't even been to synagogue since my bat mitzvah twelve years before.

"I NEED A RABBI!" she screamed, turning her head to face me, but seeming to stare right through me, her lifeless eyes shooting daggers through my heart.

I slowly backed away and melted into the bench beside her bed, simply watching things happen around me, trying to remain invisible. During the next few hours, nurses and doctors came and went. They were trying to figure out why she was so sick, but they didn't have any answers for us. We were told they were running tests. That was it. We didn't get any other information.

Later that morning, Hannah met me at the hospital, accompanied by her mom, Noreen. Noreen was the director of our Hebrew school and was the closest we would get to a rabbi. She knew exactly the types of prayers Mom needed to hear. I had never realized what an angel Noreen was until that day. Since Hannah and I had been friends for so long, Noreen had come to be another maternal figure in my life. It was comforting to have her there.

Without hesitation, Noreen sat down on Mom's bedside, held her hand, and started to sing the prayer. The moment she started to sing, Mom immediately began to relax. It was all I could

How's Your Mom?

do to watch. When Hannah's mom took a tiny pause from singing to glance around at all the nurses and people in the room, Mom begged her to continue. Somehow, that prayer was strong enough to make her feel better.

~~*~*~*~*

Finally, around mid-afternoon, the doctors seemed to acknowledge the fact that something was very, very wrong. They moved Mom downstairs, into the ICU, then almost immediately told my family that she had C. diff, a serious infection of the gut. They handed us yellow gowns, gloves, and masks, and told us to put them on right away before we could see her again. *Good thing we were just holding her hand five minutes ago,* I thought to myself but didn't dare say it out loud.

Since she was in the ICU now, only two people could visit with her at a time. This meant that Alex, Dad, and I could not all visit her at once.

We took turns for a few hours staying with her while the doctors ran more tests. Dad and I were on our way to the waiting room, in the middle of stripping off our yellow gowns, and Alex was headed in, having just put on his gloves, when suddenly a doctor appeared in our paths. She extended her hand to greet us.

"Hi, I'm Dr. Ann." She was soft-spoken, with a sympathetic face, and pretty brown curls in her hair. She was shorter than I was, and I could tell right away how seriously she took her job. I decided immediately that I liked her.

"Hi," we responded as we shook her hand, glove to glove. We formed in a circle around her sides.

"Are you the family?" she asked.

"Yeah, I'm her husband," my father said, "and these are our kids, Alex and Michelle."

"Hi," she said again. "So, we are going to give her antibiotics. She is very sick and very weak. Right now, her body is in sepsis. We know she has an infection and typically it would require surgery at this point. However, we think she is too weak. If we operate on her, there is a very high chance that she won't survive."

We nodded as if this was all completely understandable

and fine.

"So instead of operating, we will put her on antibiotics for twenty-four hours and reconsider operating tomorrow."

We nodded our heads in unison because we really had no idea what to say. We parted ways, and I instantly began replaying the conversation in my head over and over. *Too sick to operate? She might die?*

Dr. Ann walked away as Dad and I continued removing our gloves, and Alex continued putting his on. We stalled for a few moments, collaboratively digesting the information we had been given. After a few moments, Dr. Ann came back.

"Actually," she said, "we need to operate now."

We stood there, stunned.

"I'm afraid we don't have any choice," she tried to explain.

Did she really tell me that they were going to operate on her right now, despite the fact that she had JUST told me that if they operated on her, she would die? Was I hearing this correctly?

"Chris, we will need you to sign some paperwork," Dr. Ann continued. Mom had granted him her power of attorney a few years ago when she first started getting sick. She had signed a DNR. She didn't want someone to bring her back to this life if she had the chance to die. Yet, to do the surgery and potentially save her life, Dad would need to revoke the DNR so she could be intubated.

"Okay," he responded, then took the clipboard and pen in his hand. He held the pen in the air, then looked back and forth between Alex, me, and the form that would revoke her DNR. Should he allow her to be intubated? Should he try to save her, even though he knew she didn't want to live like this? Was this his chance to let her go? Was this what she wanted—a chance to be set free? Or was this just a hiccup that she shouldn't have to die from?

Moments ticked by as the pen in Dad's hand hung in the air. We all looked around at each other blankly, none of us knowing what to do. The call was Dad's to make.

CHAPTER THIRTY-FOUR
CHRIS

Everyone looked at me, and I didn't know what to do. My sister, Trudy, approached my side, and after reading the form in front of me, tried to encourage me to let her go.

"Don't sign it," she suggested. She loved Tammy as if she were her own sister, but she knew that Tammy wanted to be let go. "It's okay, Chris," she cooed the way big sisters do. "It won't be your fault."

I heard her, but I didn't listen to her. I couldn't let my baby go.

Like a magnet, my hand moved toward the paper, and I signed my name.

I should have let her go. But I couldn't. It was like when I asked her to marry me. I couldn't let her get away.

I revoked her DNR and let those doctors cut her open. I let her have another chance at living the horrible, shitty life that she desperately wanted to escape from.

I couldn't let her go.

CHAPTER THIRTY-FIVE
MICHELLE

With the paperwork signed, the ICU staff made a brief exception to the two-visitor rule so Dad, Alex, and I could have a moment together with her before they prepped her for surgery. As we said our good-byes and well wishes, she still sounded insane.

She was suddenly very concerned that Christine, who had been dating Alex for nine years, wasn't Jewish. This wasn't something she had ever told any of us before. We hadn't even known she cared much about it. I guessed it was because children are given the religion of the mother, not the father. So she didn't mind that Tyler wasn't Jewish because our kids still would be. However, if Alex and Christine had kids, they wouldn't be Jewish unless Christine converted.

"CHRISTINE!" my mother screamed. Christine wasn't even in the room.

Alex didn't say anything; he just watched, mystified, mortified, terrified, and confused, all at the same time.

"CONVERT," she yelled at the air.

We didn't respond. We let the silence suck the air out of the room.

"Have to burp . . . can't burp," she said. "HAVE TO BURP!" she said, louder this time. "CAN'T BURP! Have to burp . . ." She paused. "Can't burp."

She repeated it over and over again, sounding more like a very broken record, and nothing like Mom.

I leaned in close and held her hand tightly. "I love you, Mom," I cried softly in her ear.

When she didn't respond, I shook her hand and repeated myself again, a little louder. "Mom, I love you! Can you hear me?" My voice was on fire, burning with fear.

"DON'T SHAKE MY HAND!" she yelled at me in response.

I immediately let go of her hand and stepped back, mortified by the monster in front of me.

"Johnny . . . you make it happen," she said. Johnny was Alex's best friend, who happened to be Jewish, and Mom must have thought he held the power to make Christine want to convert. He wasn't in the room, either.

I took a step forward again, now agitated and completely terrified about the fact that this might be the last conversation we'd ever have.

"MOM!" I screamed in her ear. "I LOVE YOU, CAN YOU HEAR ME?"

She stared at the ceiling, her hand laying lifeless in mine. "Have to burp . . . can't burp."

My heart raced, and my chest felt like it was going to explode. *WHERE DID MOM GO?*

I wondered if this was the end. Was this the last time I was going to see her? Would the last thing on her mind before she died be about having to burp?

"MOM! ANSWER ME!"

I looked longingly at Dad, desperate for him to fix her. He looked back at me sympathetically, then wiped his tears with the back of his glove-covered hand.

"Tammy, baby," he said lightly, staring through her eyes as if trying to reach her soul.

She didn't hear him. She just kept yelling things at everyone in the room and everyone not in the room. Her broken phrases made no sense. "CHRIS!" "CONVERT!" "JOHNNY!"

Her screams grew louder with every passing minute. Everyone in the ICU could hear her.

I looked at Alex, who had been standing silent and still as a statue the entire time. There was a tear on his cheek. It was the first time I had ever, in our entire lives, seen him cry. *Yeah, this was bad.*

Simultaneously, the three of us wiped our tears and then took turns kissing Mom on her cheek. She was there, in front of us, but she was gone. She was so far gone.

And that was the end. We took off our gloves, gowns, and masks, and headed to the waiting room. It was ten o'clock at night.

CHAPTER THIRTY-SIX

MICHELLE

I mean, that was the end. That *had* to be the end.

I knew how sick she was. I knew Mom better than anyone. I knew she hated having MS, and I knew she was absolutely incredibly weak, and I knew, in the depths of my heart, that she wouldn't survive that surgery. I was absolutely sure of it.

I spent the entire night with my stomach in knots, crying constantly. A steady stream of never-ending tears poured from my eyes all night long. A lot of our family and friends had shown up to be with us, and, sensing that we had a long night ahead of us, I asked Tyler to escort me to Dunkin Donuts so we could get some coffee and munchies for everyone. As I placed our order, the tears kept flowing. I ignored them, letting them fall from my face onto the counter in front of me, not even bothering to wipe them away or hide them from the confused teenaged cashier who was staring at me. I figured that I might as well wear on my sleeve the pain that was destroying me inside.

When we returned to the ICU, Dad stood up and said, "Congratulations!" I was so confused. I looked at Tyler, whose eyes grew so wide I thought he had seen a ghost.

"For what?" I asked, completely confused, looking back and forth from Dad to Tyler.

Dad looked at Tyler and must have realized something. "For, uh, living!" Dad said quickly, then sat immediately back down. He picked up a magazine and began to flip through the pages . . . clearly trying to move on.

Had Tyler been planning to propose? I wondered with butterflies aggressively filling my stomach. *Oh, Dad. What did you just do?*

For Tyler's sake, I decided to let the whole thing go. I walked to the other side of the room and sat down like I was completely clueless, and stayed as far away from Mr. Big Mouth as I could.

As we waited in the ICU waiting room for what felt like an eternity, all I could do was cry. My cousins talked and told stories to try to keep us all distracted. I appreciated their efforts, but it didn't really make a difference. Nothing would be able to stop the tears. She was going to die. She was probably already dead. The longer the surgery took, the surer I became.

Hours rolled by with no updates.

First, it was midnight, then one o'clock, then two. Finally, around four o'clock, Dr. Ann cracked open the waiting room door, the only thing separating us from the unknown.

"Hi," she said softly as she stepped into the room, closing the door gently behind her while removing her gloves. "Can you all come over here?" My family was scattered around the waiting room, and some friends were waiting outside in the surrounding hallways. Immediately, we all jumped to our feet and congregated around her.

"She survived," she informed us. We collectively let out an audible sigh of relief.

"Her infection was in her large intestine. We had to remove a large piece of it. She had a colectomy." I had no idea what any of this meant, or what the implications would be, nor did I care. I was too in awe. There were no words for how I felt at that moment.

We wouldn't be able to see her that night, so the surgeon told us all to go home, get some rest, and come back to visit her in the morning. Dad shook her hand, thanked her for saving his wife's life, and wiped tears from his face.

As we pulled into the driveway, I couldn't help thinking, *Home again, home again, jiggity jig.* Even though it was almost five a.m., we were all too hyped up to sleep. We needed vodka, we decided. Happily, Dad poured Tyler, himself, and me a shot of Grey Goose. We clinked our glasses in celebration of Tammy, the ultimate fighter.

--*-*-*-*

We awoke feeling optimistic and refreshed. We each ate a filling breakfast of eggs, home fries, and bacon, and took our time getting ready. It was the first full meal Dad had eaten all week. Our spirits were high. Then Dad's cell phone rang.

It was the anesthesiologist, calling to tell us that Mom's

body wasn't responding to anything. That her kidneys were shutting down and her blood pressure was too low. That we should get to her as soon as possible.

We rushed to the hospital to find Mom, bloated, seemingly unconscious and hooked up to three separate IV carts, a total of twelve IVs. The tears immediately began again. She wasn't awake. She wasn't responding to anything we said to her. Could she hear us? If it weren't for the steady beeps of the life support machine, I would have sworn she wasn't really alive. How could this happen overnight?

We spoke directly into her ear, thinking that was the only way we could get her to hear us. *Mom? Can you hear me? It's okay. You're going to fight. Mom?* Over and over, we repeated in her ear, *we love you. We love you. We love you. We love you.*

Before we knew it, our entire family seemed to show up again. They all had to drive hours to get to the hospital, and it just hit me that they were coming to say good-bye. This was it; she wasn't going to make it. There was no way. She was too weak. Her body couldn't take any more.

Hannah showed up to the hospital, and I cried to her. I told her I didn't want to lose Mom. That I wasn't just losing her today, but that she would be gone forever, and that I still had so many questions to ask her. I needed to learn how to cook. I wanted to learn more about our distant relatives and understand the relationships better. I want to know how to use kitchen gadgets. How do you get a ring out of a coffee table? How do you plan a wedding?

Then I realized that my mother wouldn't be at my wedding. That she wouldn't meet her grandchildren. She was going to miss so much.

I started to miss her. I missed Mom so much, and I begged my best friend for Mom not to die. I cried until I found the strength to pause, and then Hannah walked with me back upstairs to join the rest of my family.

When we walked upstairs, we were immediately greeted by Noreen. She wrapped me in a warm embrace, instantly causing my tears to begin again, then pulled Hannah in for a group hug. She held us and told me that none of this would be easy, but that she would help answer my questions. She assured me that Mom was so loved, and she wasn't gone yet, but that if Mom did need to go away, I would be okay.

I loved her, and I was so grateful for her kindness. But I didn't believe her when she said I would be okay. I wouldn't. She couldn't answer my questions; only Mom could. Mom was my best friend. No one was ever going to replace her. Nothing about losing her would be okay.

As the day went on, everyone got a chance to visit Mom's bedside. Everyone who entered needed to wear gowns and gloves because her infection was still contagious. In between visits, the nurses would check her vitals, rotate her body, and pump her medicines. We ate lunch and then heard her kidneys were beginning to work, and for the first time all day, we had hope.

Sometime in the mid-afternoon, Dad and I were able to see her again. We hadn't seen her since the morning because of the two-person rule, and there were hours' worth of visitors. But this time, when we saw her, she was able to nod her head. She could furrow her brow, and I swore I saw tears in the corner of her eyes. I told her that Noreen couldn't answer my questions and that I needed her to fight. I begged her to stay. Dad begged her to stay. And she heard us. I knew she did.

Feeling slightly refreshed, we kissed her forehead and left the room to give others a chance to be with her. By dinner time, she was really getting better. And there was no real explanation for it.

Around eight that night, we asked the nurses for an update. They said we should go home, that things were looking hopeful, and that Mom really just needed to sleep. We understood but wanted to say goodnight to her. We quickly went into her cubicle and found her eyes wide open, bugged-eyed. It still didn't appear that she could hear us or respond to us, but at least her eyes were open. She might have still been comatose, but surely opening her eyes was a sign of great progress. The only thing we were still unsure of was whether or not her brain had been damaged. The lights might have been on, but was anyone home? Was everything still functioning the way it should have?

"Mom," I said. "I'm so glad you're still here."

"Blink once if you're okay," Dad instructed. I held my breath. If she could hear him and understand his request, then we would know that the lights were on *and* somebody was home.

Without missing a beat, she blinked.

CHAPTER THIRTY-SEVEN
CHRIS

Being in the ICU with her was horrible. I was there from morning to night every day. I ate every meal (well, the ones I remembered to eat) in the hospital cafeteria. I worried about our dog because there was no one to let her out.

Tammy had twelve IVs and a breathing tube. I counted them.

At one point, I stopped in at the financial office to see what the damage was. She had been in the ICU for three days so far, and the price tag was forty-eight thousand dollars per day. I had no idea how I would pay for it, and I didn't have the mental capacity to try to figure it out, either.

Tammy and I had taken out ten-year life insurance policies before her official diagnosis. Her policy was worth $500,000. At the very least, I knew that if she died, her life insurance would pay the medical bills. But if she didn't die, I didn't know what I would do.

Then again, I didn't know what I would if she *did* die, either.

I had two fears pressing on my mind and heart that week: that I would lose my wife of over thirty years, and that I would go into extreme amounts of debt. Each fear seemed to be the solution for the other.

I couldn't solve any of those problems that week. It was all I could do to remember to eat food sometimes, and spend all my remaining energy praying that the doctors would be able to remove her breathing tube. The sooner they removed the breathing tube, the sooner she could be released from the ICU and moved upstairs into a room. Of course, I wanted her out of the ICU because of how expensive it was.

But how could I even begin to think about paying all of this off, when we didn't know if she would ever wake up?

CHAPTER THIRTY-EIGHT

MICHELLE

Over the course of the first three days in the ICU, we saw Mom making some great progress, but she still wasn't waking up. She was comatose, and all I wanted was to hug her and talk to her. I was grateful that her kidneys began producing output and she was able to come completely off her blood pressure medicines. Still, I missed her. I wanted her to look at me and hear me. I understood there was a lot to be happy about, but there was a lot to be sad about, too.

Some nights were difficult to fall asleep. I couldn't get her out of my head. I kept seeing her in her delusional state before surgery. I heard her loud, chaotic screams . . .

Have to burp . . . Can't burp . . .
Hebrew school. Jewish. Convert.
CHRISTINE! Johnny, you make it happen.
DON'T SHAKE MY HAND. MICHELLLLLLE!

I pictured her wide-open eyes, dilated pupils, and tears spilling out as Dad asked if she liked the sound of his voice. I saw her nod. I thought of her skin, so bloated and stretched to the brim. Her hand that looked like a boxing glove.

I thought of the future and wondered what each coming day would be like. What would happen in a week? I found myself losing my breath, breathing uncontrollably hard and feeling like I couldn't calm down.

˷˷*˷*˷*

On day four, our family met in the ICU waiting room to try to figure out what our plan would be. How long would we keep her on life support? How long would we keep her alive if she didn't wake up? We knew she wouldn't want a feeding bag, and that seemed to be the place where we would draw the line. But how long would we wait for her to wake up?

The thing was, I could hear her in my head. I kept hearing her say *let me try to fight, but don't force me if I can't.* It was like she was telling me to give her a shot and see how she did, but not to force her if she didn't want to fight anymore.

"Dad, I think we should give her a little more time to fight it," I had suggested on day three.

"You're right," he said, then told the doctors that we decided we should keep the breathing tube in for one more day.

On day four, they removed her breathing tube without any issues. She didn't even flinch when they pulled it out. She could cough, swallow, and open her eyes when she was in pain. Other than that, she still didn't respond to much. But her lungs and heart were working perfectly fine.

After the breathing tube came out, Dad, Alex, and I spent some time talking with her and giving her the latest updates. Then Tyler and I sat in the waiting room for a while, while Dad continued to visit with Mom and begged her to come back to us. In the afternoons, her friends would visit.

By day five, we were desperate for her to open her eyes again. She hadn't opened them again the night when she'd been completely bug-eyed and unresponsive, and I still wasn't sure if there was anyone home inside her head. I begged her, shook her, poked her, yelled loudly in her ear while my tears fell on her gown. Her eyes remained glued shut, her body still as a statue. Dad kissed her face and cried on her and begged her to show us that she was still in there somewhere. She didn't.

Dad liked to make sure that Mom's lips weren't chapped, so he applied a ton of Chapstick and constantly wet them with a little sponge. She bit down on the mouth sponge so firmly, and that Dad couldn't pull it out of her mouth. We figured that meant she wanted cake—her absolute favorite food.

I yelled to the nurse. "Why can she use so much energy to bite down on the mouth sponge but she can't even open her eyes? Doesn't it require more energy to bite than to flick open your eyes?" The nurse politely informed me that biting was an involuntary, natural reaction. Opening her eyes was something we were asking her to do. *You're telling me she is probably brain dead,* I thought. Again, I cried.

I swore that I heard her while I was standing over her, screaming at her to wake up. I could hear her saying, *I'm so tired, Michelle. I'm sorry. I'm just so tired. . . .* and then she sort of drifted off the way she usually did when she was tired from MS fatigue. She placed a lot of emphasis on the *tiiiiiiii-red. So tiiiii-red.* That's what she used to say so often.

Each night, I sat with Dad in our living room at our home, alternating between acting like everything was fine and having complete meltdowns. Dad kept asking if he should have any regrets. Should he have let her have the shoulder surgery? Should he have let the doctors cut her open again when she was infected? Could he have taken better care of her? Did he yell at her too much? Was he patient enough with her? I needed to keep reminding him that he was the best caregiver Mom could have ever had and that she appreciated him so much. I reminded him that he should have no regrets at all, and he repeated back, "No regrets. I need to keep reminding myself of that."

I knew that Mom knew how lucky she was because she always said she would be "up shit's creek without him." She always said he took such good care of her that she forgot she was sick. I reminded Dad of this, and he replied that he hadn't ever heard her say that. Honestly, he didn't ever listen. She said it all the time.

I looked at Mom's empty chair, and I felt another pang of missing her. I looked through her iPad and found a note that she'd written and, again, could feel her talking to me. One note contained a list of all our family members, with a total count of sixty-one at the bottom of the page. *Why did she write this?* I wondered. And then it hit me: She'd made it for my wedding. She must have thought that a proposal was coming. She knew I'd need help with the guest list.

I missed her so much. I cried, and it felt like it was never going to stop. Dad headed off to bed, thanked me for "helping," and said "I love you so much. I love you long time."

I told him, "I love you long time," in my strangest Indian-sounding accent. Not sure why, but that's how we always said it.

Before I fell asleep that night, I prayed that she would open

How's Your Mom?

her eyes to tell us she loved us just one more time. *Please, Mom. I need to really listen when you say it this time.*

CHAPTER THIRTY-NINE

MICHELLE

As I had grappled with the fear of losing Mom all week, I noticed myself having a completely different view on everything in the world. I noticed the elderly and found myself being jealous of all the little old ladies who'd had the chance to grow old. I wondered about their life stories—did they have daughters? Grandkids? Were they perfectly healthy or sick, too? How old would they get to grow? Why did they get to grow old and Mom didn't? What had they done differently?

At one point, I caught myself staring at a girl about my age, sitting with her mom in the hospital cafeteria. They were having a perfectly normal conversation, but to me, that conversation was everything. I wanted to walk over to them and tell them how lucky they were. I wanted to offer to take a picture of them so they would always remember that moment, that conversation, and realize how fortunate they were. Instead, I clutched at my chest, turned away, and realized I would never get to have a conversation with Mom again.

In my journey to the cafeteria that day, I found myself getting lost in the hallways, and I wasn't even surprised I was lost. I thought, *of course, I'm lost. I don't have a mom anymore. I'll probably always be lost.*

I felt independent in a way I never had felt before, in a way I'd never wanted to have to feel. I wondered as a cashier took three dollars for my coffee if she could tell how broken I was. Was it obvious to everyone? Did I suddenly look like a girl who'd lost her mom?

Mostly, I just missed her. I felt her everywhere I went. I heard her in my head and felt her presence all around me in every single thing I did.

I was broken. I couldn't look people in the eye, couldn't stop feeling sorry for myself, for my family. I wondered if anyone else in that hospital hurt as much as I was.

No, I decided. No one was as broken as I was.

~~*~*~*~*

By day six in the ICU, Mom was able to keep her eyes open all day and was doing things like licking her lips, moving her jaw, and continuing to suck on the sponge filled with water that I put in her mouth. She was acting as if she were awake, but she was still comatose. Although her eyes were open and she seemed responsive, she wasn't able to really look at us or speak to us. It was like she was only half-awake. It was scary as hell.

I begged our doctor to consult with a neurologist to assure us that everything was still working in her brain. No neurologists never showed up, but I didn't mind. Dad and I just sat with her all day. I laid down beside her and talked to her, telling her all the things I had always wanted to say, reminding her of all our good memories together, and told her everyone who was thinking about her. She didn't respond to me, but I told myself she could hear me. When I played our song, "I Hope You Dance" for her, her eyes lit up, and she caught her breath. Sure, it could have been a coincidence that she just randomly caught her breath, but I was pretty sure that she recognized our song. Maybe her brain wasn't dead.

Tyler came to see her around seven that night, and he swore she looked at him when he walked in. Another great sign.

I had been with her for twelve hours that day, and I was so content that when I got home, for the first time all week, I didn't feel the urge to cry. It didn't take long for me to fall asleep and I slept soundly through the night.

The next morning, I took my time getting ready for the day, unsure whether or not I would actually make it into work. As I strolled aimlessly around my kitchen and tried to plan my day, my cell phone rang.

"Hello?" I answered. It was Christine, who had stopped by the hospital on her way to work.

"Your mom wants you," she told me.

"What?" I obviously hadn't heard her right. How could Mom want me if she was partially comatose?

"She's responsive now," Christine continued. "You're the

only one who can fix her pillows the right way. She needs you to come right now."

"Oh my gosh. I'm on my way." I hung up the phone and flew out the door, sped down Main Street, and sprinted to her room in the ICU.

"Michelle. . . ." Mom's voice was scratchy and weak, but it didn't matter. She was saying my name. She was looking at me, and hearing me, and speaking directly to me. She was out of her coma.

I was drawn to her like a magnet, instantly planting my head on her chest and wrapping my arms around her body. Mom was awake and completely aware. She moved her head an inch to rest it on top of mine, her best attempt at a hug, as she was unable to move anything else.

MS had, once again, tried to take everything it could away from her.

But Mom had *won*.

This is what a miracle feels like.

CHAPTER FORTY

TAMMY

A mother's perspective: Firsts.

We had done other "firsts" before. First day of preschool. First school bus ride to Charlotte Avenue Elementary School. First day of dance class. First bat mitzvah party. First day of overnight camp. First day at Nashua High School. But this was the first dorm move-in day.

I fought back my own memories of my first day of college. I tried to keep from comparing it to move-in day of her older brother. This was HER day. But here we were, big brother, Mom, and Michelle dutifully toting the items to her room that would serve her creature comforts for her first year of dorm life.

We had always been like the llama in Dr. Doolittle. We had a *push-me— pull-you* relationship where she was pointed in the opposite direction from me. Always pulling, not allowing me to lead. Yet we were connected, and I felt her need to remain a part of me.

I can do it myself, Mom! she would say.

Let me show you first, child, I would think.

She was so different from me in my naivete, but so like me in my desire to show Mom that I could make it in the world without her.

We had done all the college tours. I, in the role of good mother, tried to take her to a variety of campuses. We toured Johnson and Wales in Providence, Rhode Island. We had a lovely trip to Roger Williams University. We chose the coldest day of the year to walk around the University of Massachusetts Amherst. We toured the University of New Hampshire.

The big campuses were beautiful. You could feel college life pulsating around you. Dreams and hopes, energy and youth vibrated from every building. I wanted her to see what money could buy. I wanted her to know that her education was important and I, as her parent, was encouraging her to make her own choice. After each visit, I would ask her if it felt right. Were those the kind of people she wished to associate with? Money can buy anything in life, but is that the kind of life you want to live?

I told her that she owed it to herself, and to me, as a New Hampshire resident, to visit New Hampshire's only state college. We had nothing to lose, and there was always a nice breakfast offering at these events. Michelle did not see the point of even visiting the one place she knew she would not attend. "There's nothing there for me. I want to go to a university with a true college experience," was her battle cry.

We finally took the obligatory tour of Keene State College. At Keene, my petulant daughter kept an attitude of distant skepticism. Our first step on campus, we were greeted by a woman who, based on her appearance, we guessed to be a professor. She smiled and offered direction and wished us a good day. *Hmm, friendly people here,* I thought. The tour of the campus yielded an atmosphere only found in New Hampshire. The late winter day was cold, the sun was warm. The buildings were modern, the people were down-to-earth. But it was the presentation of the academics of the college that caught Michelle's attention. The program appealed to her. She related to the course offerings and the philosophy of the college's education plan.

"I wasn't supposed to like it here," she said.

And I smiled and felt the relief only a mother can feel when she knows her child has found the place to take her first steps into this big scary world.

Over the summer, we shopped. I tried to think of everything that would keep my baby girl comfortable. Towels and pillows, lamps, and desk accessories, posters, shower caddy, trash basket, snacks, silverware, pencil sharpener, laptop . . . the list danced before my eyes. It kept me up at night. I didn't want to forget anything. I wanted her to be comfortable.

That fall, we schlepped it all into her dorm room at Keddy Hall. As a mother, I was calmed by this building. It was small. Her first experience away from home would not be in one of those crazy dorms. I noted the security of the building and her room. Locks, fire extinguishers. Her physical safety could be assured.

We met her roommate and her family. I liked them. Her roommate's mom gave the girls gifts. I sensed the *push-me—pull-you* relationship that they, too, shared and I prayed these girls would find their own place in the world. We discussed furniture arrangement and poster placement. We set up her laundry hamper. We stowed her snacks. I made her bed and hid our book in the bed caddy. Her physical comfort was assured.

I wanted her to choreograph her own dance as she journeyed forward into life. I wanted the steps to hold echoes of her past only going forward while remembering the steps she had already traveled.

What was next? There was supposed to be a meeting for the new honor society students. Where was it to be held? I had not paid attention to the instructions when we first entered. I was too concerned with Michelle's physical safety and comfort. I suppose I already expected that Michelle would take responsibility for the rest. But we did not know where to go for that meeting. Where had everyone disappeared to? Why did they all know where to go, but we did not? We went outside. No one was around. We walked down the street, rushing now, searching for where we were supposed to be.

We asked a man in a kitchen uniform if he knew anything about the meeting. Yes, he told us, there would be a barbeque later for the new dorm students. We were still unsure where Michelle should be at that moment. We went back to Keddy Hall, hoping to find someone to direct us. We found another mother who pointed the way. The students were in a room down the hall. The meeting had already started, which meant Michelle would have to walk into the room with everyone watching her. No graceful, inconspicuous entrance here!

The tears began. This was suddenly too much to handle. It was all too new. Uncertainty crept in. The desire to go home cried out.

There were never tears at any of the other firsts. Through my own tears, I hugged her and pushed her away at the same time. I whispered in her ear, "You can do this, Michelle. You can walk into that room. You will find your place." I hoped my words would soothe her as she began her journey into a new life without me.

CHAPTER FORTY-ONE

MICHELLE

While all of the chaos was unfolding at the hospital, I did all I could to feel normal. Dad, Alex, extended family members, and I had climbed up and down the scale of uncertainty far too often over the past few weeks, having no idea what would happen with Mom. Around day four in the ICU, my cousin, Jen, offered me the most useful advice I'd ever gotten: "Stay at a five," she told me. "You'll get good news, and you'll shoot up to a ten, and then something will set it back, and you'll fall to a zero," she explained. "It's too much, and it makes things too hard to handle."

So I tried to remain at a level five. If I stayed at a five, no matter what news I received, then I might be able to handle everything that was happening with a few less emotional outbursts.

It worked for a little while.

On the same day that Mom had spoken my name for the first time all week, the doctors decided we could transfer her to a regular room upstairs. We were so grateful to get her out of that ICU. It was a Friday night, and Tyler had just shown up at the hospital. We would wait upstairs for Mom to arrive.

We sat on the bench in the dimly lit room with my cousin, Sarah, who had also arrived to visit. We made idle conversation and waited patiently for Mom to arrive. It felt like hours had passed. A few people came into the room and introduced themselves to me. They would be Mom's nurses. I was relieved they all seemed so nice, and I silently prayed that they would each take good care of her.

Finally, Mom was wheeled into her new room. Sarah leapt to her feet to give her a big hug, then remained standing by her bedside. I joined Sarah, both of us looking admiringly down at Mom. She smiled back at both of us.

"Is there any cake up here?" she asked as nurses rolled her bed into the perfect spot. *She's really back,* I thought to myself.

Sarah and I laughed together and looked over our shoulders as if a cake would actually appear on the counter behind us.

"We'll bake you a cake when you go home," I offered sincerely.

Tyler had been quietly sitting on the bench beside us, until suddenly, he shot up to his feet. "There's something I've been wanting to ask you," he said to me. I turned around to face him as Sarah immediately reached for her cell phone camera, and Tyler reached for my hand. "I need to ask you now."

Before I knew it, he was down on one knee, showing me a beautiful "Hearts on Fire" diamond ring. The band was sterling silver with tiny twists on each side, and there was a round diamond in the center that sparkled up at me.

I giggled nervously, then instantly asked, "Really? Right now?"

He nodded. "Will you marry me?"

Tyler and I had been dating for over six years at that point. I had pictured, over the past few years, all of the ways I thought he would propose to me: on the quad at Keene State College, at the house where we first met, on the top of Mount Monadnock (the mountain we used to hike in the fall that was twenty minutes from campus), on the day we moved into our first apartment together. Each of those events came and went without a proposal, and each time I was surer he was planning his proposal for just the right time.

I looked down at him, still smiling, but the smile didn't feel as genuine as I wanted it to. I couldn't believe this would be our proposal story for the rest of our lives. Now, every time I told the story, I would have to start with *"Well, we were in the hospital. . . . and Mom had just come out of a coma . . . because she had MS . . . and she fell out of her wheelchair. . . . which was my fault . . ."*

I shoved the thoughts out of my mind. "YES!" I exclaimed in a high-pitched squeak, the voice I used only when I was being fake. "Gimmie, gimmie, gimmie!" I greedily reached for the shiny diamond in front of me and pulled him up to standing. I hated myself for reacting that way, but I blamed the circumstances and the fact that I had absolutely no idea what to do or say.

How's Your Mom?

He slipped it effortlessly onto my left ring finger. The ring was way too big, but I pretended like it wasn't. I took a step backwards and thrust my left hand in Mom's face while pinching it with my other fingers, so I didn't accidentally fling it off. "LOOK!"

"Wow . . ." she croaked. "Congratulations." She was weak; her energy had not yet returned.

Within moments, a crowd of nurses appeared in the room, offering their congratulations and asking to see the ring. I showed it off, as I knew Tyler would want me to, but I was afraid to admit what I was thinking out loud: *I can't believe that's how he proposed.*

I found out a week later that Tyler had planned to propose to me the night Mom was admitted to the ICU. He had asked Dad for permission that morning, which explained the random *congratulations for living* comment that Dad had made. Dad must have thought that Tyler would still propose that night. *Oh, Dad.*

One of my favorite events of the year was taking place that night Mom was admitted—the Nashua Holiday Stroll. At the top of Main Street, a giant Christmas tree would be lit, and thousands of people would congregate to watch the lighting and then stroll down Main Street. Almost every year since we had started dating, Tyler had come to the Holiday Stroll with me, and we had taken a picture in front of the tree. His plan was to drop to one knee as we were taking this annual picture. Instead, he stayed with me and many of my extended family members in the ICU waiting room.

That was the thing about dating a girl whose mom had MS. You couldn't actually plan on anything. The villain didn't just steal from the person who had it—it stole from everyone around them, too.

˯˯*˯*˯*˯*

Later that night, Sarah and I drove back to my parents' house as Tyler followed in his car behind us.

"So, do you like the ring?" Sarah asked me.

The truth was that I didn't like the ring. I wanted the band to have smaller diamonds on each side, or at least a little bit of sparkle. The band was too plain. The diamond was pretty, but he told me that you needed to look under a microscope to see the "hearts on fire" effect. Apparently, it looked like the diamond was on fire or something when you shined a light through it the right way. The salesman had shown Tyler in the store, but I would probably never get to see it myself since the diamond was already set on the ring. I knew he'd tried to pick out the perfect ring, but the truth was that I didn't like it at all. I couldn't help the way I felt.

I also didn't like the way he had proposed. I was so happy that Mom was alive. . . . but I could not believe that he asked me the very same day she woke up.

"No," I confessed. "I don't like the band. And I can't believe he picked today to ask me. What was he thinking?" I looked longingly at Sarah as she drove ahead.

"Maybe he was thinking that he loved you, wanted to marry you, and knew you would want your mom to be there for the proposal," Sarah offered.

"I mean, yeah, but . . ." I threw my hands up at my sides in a way that I hoped conveyed what I was feeling: *WHAT THE FUCK!*

"I know," she said. "It's not what you expected."

"None of this is what I expected," I told her angrily. My teeth chattered, a sign that always told me I was upset, even when I didn't want to admit it. But I was furious and only comforted by the fact that I knew I didn't need to hold back when I was with Sarah. "Now am I supposed to call my friends and family with the news and sound happy? How am I supposed to be happy right now? That was the WORST proposal ever," I yelled at the air, then paused to breathe. "I thought I was supposed to stay at a five . . . How am I going to stay at a five right now? ARE YOU KIDDING ME?" I slapped my hands down on the seat beside me, my entire body shaking.

"I know, you must be feeling pretty conflicted right now. But think of it this way," Sarah said calmly. "This morning, you didn't even know if your mom was going to survive. And now, your mom is alive, and you are marrying Tyler."

I couldn't help but smile at that realization. When she put it that way, it didn't sound so terrible. Suddenly, I realized how very brave Tyler had been by asking me when he did.

I wondered how different my reaction would have been if he had been able to ask me at the Holiday Stroll. For the millionth time, I couldn't help thinking *damn you, MS. You ruin every single thing.*

"But don't you think it's kind of cool that he fully committed himself to you during the most challenging time of your life?" Sarah continued. "Hopefully, you'll never have to go through anything as horrible as this ever again. But if you do, you'll know for sure that Tyler will be by your side, no matter what."

"Well, I hadn't thought about it that way," I admitted.

"Michelle, it's amazing. Seriously, you and Tyler are so lucky to have each other."

She was right. It *was* amazing. I thought about how he had stood by me all week long while I waited for Mom to wake up. I thought of all the moments over the course of the week where he let me literally cry on his shoulder, yell at him, and sit in silence with him. I had apologized profusely for acting like such a lunatic, and he told me it was okay over and over again. He understood. He had never *not* been there when I needed him to be, and now I knew that would be the case for the rest of our lives.

I really was pretty lucky.

And, in addition, Mom had been able to witness one of the greatest moments in my life.

At the start of that car ride, I had been furiously thinking about how fucking MS ruined absolutely every good thing in my life. But by the time we pulled into our driveway, I realized it was okay that the proposal wasn't how I had planned. I accepted the fact that nothing ever went as planned anyway. *When man plans, G-d laughs,* I heard Mom tell me in my head, as she had so many times before. I was not only optimistic about the great volumes of love the proposal represented but actually grateful that it happened the way it did. It allowed me to see how much Tyler really loved me. We didn't need any pomp and circumstance. I could already tell, by his actions, that he loved me.

When I realized how much my perspective changed during

that short car ride, I couldn't help but think that Mom wasn't the only one who had beaten MS that day.

I realized that MS was simply a test of how well you could change your perspective. When MS is in your life, you absolutely needed to have a flexible perspective. That was it.

For the first time in my life, I had *finally* beaten MS, too.

Mother-daughter team for the win.

PART FOUR
MOVING IN
December 2015–August 2017

CHAPTER FORTY-TWO

TAMMY

Home again, home again, jiggity jig.

The first thing I noticed when I was brought into my bedroom after those long weeks in the hospital was my new hospital bed. After thirty-one years of marriage and cuddling with my husband, we were relegated to separate beds.

And if that didn't cut short the romance, my husband would now be the primary person taking care of my poop bag.

I learned that after certain hospital stays, you get a visiting nurse to check on you. When my visiting nurse came, I confessed my displeasure with my situation.

"I'm now a person with advancing MS and an ostomy bag," I cried to her. "It is completely impossible for me to take care of myself. When it was just MS, I had a chance. But my hands don't work well enough for me to be able to change this poop bag." I flailed my right hand in the air, showing her how useless it was. And that was my only working extremity.

She didn't respond.

"I don't want to live like this," I finally cried.

She told me she understood. "Well, we could see about admitting you into the hospice program."

I was intrigued.

"We would need to examine you to see if you would qualify," she explained, "but if you do, then we will be able to make sure you are comfortable."

I nodded, certain that was what I wanted. I hoped that I would be accepted. "I don't want to live like this."

The following day, another nurse decided that I was indeed eligible for hospice care. "We will provide you with all the medications relative to your condition," she told me.

"Thank you," I offered, wondering how many medications I would actually require.

"We will have a nurse come once a week, and an aide will

visit three times a week to get you cleaned up," she told me. "How does that sound?"

"That sounds very nice," I replied, dabbing what felt like constant tears from the corners of my eyes.

"The only thing you have to do is *not* seek extra care. If you decide you want to go back to a doctor or take any medications for treating your MS again, then you won't be able to stay in hospice."

Hospice would provide for me as long as I was hopeless, I thought to myself. How lucky was I? There it was again . . . hope versus despair. "As long as I'm hopeless," I told her out loud.

She laughed nervously, uncertain how to respond.

I kept thinking that it was all a bad dream and I would wake up and walk away. In reality, it was in the dream that I was walking, and in my wakeful hours that I was lying in bed unable to walk or move about.

CHAPTER FORTY-THREE
MICHELLE

We needed an angel wing.

Without an angel wing, it was very difficult to shift Mom's hips while she laid in bed. An angel wing was sort of like a sheet— it had soft fabric on one side and a slippery surface on the other. It lay across the bed like a sheet, but it had "wings" that hung over the sides. You could pull on the wings to move the person laying on top of it without actually having to touch the person. It's quite a handy invention, actually. And we needed at least one of them. It was important.

I was on a mission to use my sweetest, most charming personality to see if the nurses at the hospital where Mom had lived for the past three weeks would be willing to give us a free angel wing.

As I entered the hospital where Mom had almost died, I tried not to pay attention to the memories that instantly flooded back to me. Everything from the parking lot and the lady at the front desk to the elevator and the hallways seemed to reek of tainted memories. Had the last few weeks really happened? They all felt like a nightmare to me.

I followed the path I now had memorized through the winding hallways and up to the fifth floor where Mom had spent the last two weeks of her hospital stay. I approached the nurses' station and gazed at the nurse through the glass window. She smiled at me and slid open the glass door.

"Michelle!" she squealed in delight. I wasn't sure if she would remember me, but she did. I gave a mental high-five to nurses everywhere who cared so much about their patients and their families, without always getting a chance to realize how much their compassion really meant. It was both touching and impressive that she remembered my name. (Although it was possible that I had become known as *the girl who got engaged*, and that's why she remembered me.) Either way, I was touched.

"Hi," I said shyly back. I remembered this nurse, and I was

happy she was the one on duty. Her name was Trisha. Out of all of the nurses who had taken care of Mom, she was our favorite. She had a short blonde pixie cut and a sarcastic sense of humor. We had gotten to know each other quite well; I knew she had a pet squirrel, which she'd rescued when it was just a baby after it fell out of a tree and broke its leg. She had found it lying on the street, picked it up, brought it home, nursed it back to health, and raised it like a kitten. It was now a fully-adult squirrel that she kept as a pet. I thought it was the coolest thing.

"How are you?" she asked cautiously. Before I had a chance to answer, she continued. "How's your mom?"

"She's good," I said, unsure why I felt the desire to lie to Mom's own nurse, and my favorite nurse, at that. If anyone knew the truth, it was her. *Old habits die hard,* I thought.

We made casual small talk, which I was grateful for. I hated having to ask people for things, and I used the time we spent making small talk to work up the nerve. She knew Mom incredibly well and continued to talk about all of the ways she and Mom had laughed together over the past two weeks. It was amazing that they had actually become such good friends. Then again, Mom could befriend a tree if it let her. She was just the type of person that every living thing liked.

"So . . . do you have any questions about hospice?" she asked me kindly.

Hospice? I didn't know what she was talking about. My confusion must have shown on my face, because she continued, "Oh . . . I thought you knew. We recommended your mom be admitted into the hospice program, and I believe she was accepted."

My heart sank. I didn't have any words. Did hospice mean she was going to die? It was the program for those who were half-dead, or soon to be dead, right?

It hit me: Mom may have survived the surgery, but she was still going to die. I immediately looked down, Trisha's eye contact feeling like too much pressure to bear. Trisha must have sensed my unease and instantly began backpedaling. "It's okay!" she continued. "It's a good thing."

I forced my eyes to meet hers, and tears instantly flooded them. I think this made her feel bad because tears formed in her eyes as well. I hated when I made other people cry.

Trisha began telling me about her own experience when her mom was admitted into hospice, and how scared she had felt. She was the one who had to call an ambulance when her mom had a heart episode. Her mom also made it out of the hospital alive, but she was the only one around to take care of her. Her mom was admitted to hospice, too, and she stayed alive for six months. She put an emphasis on the *six months* like this was supposed to make me feel better.

She ended her story with tears pouring down her own face. Crying at the expense of her situation, instead of mine, allowed me to feel like it was okay to cry in front of her. *I wasn't crying for me. I was crying for her.* Or maybe, *we were both crying for each other.*

Somehow, hearing her story did make mine feel less terrifying. At the very least, it was good to know that I wasn't the only one who was afraid of the *H* word.

I didn't say much while she talked. I just listened and nodded. Sometimes, people just needed to be heard. You didn't always have to say anything back.

After she finished telling her story, she looked at me, waiting for me to respond. "Wow, six months . . . that's a long time . . ." my voice trailed, uncertain of whether she was trying to make me feel hopeful or prepared. Was that how long I would have until Mom died, too?

"I thought people were only in hospice for a little while . . . until they . . . you know . . ." again, my voice trailed.

She shook her head and explained that the purpose of hospice was to provide people with all of the care and support required to make them feel comfortable. This was a good thing, she assured me because she would have nurses who would visit the house to take care of her. She would also have access to the hospice home if she ever needed to be monitored around the clock. We were lucky she'd been admitted.

I thanked her for the information and did my best to wear

a brave face. Suddenly, my request for an angel wing didn't feel like such a big deal anymore. It's funny how disease makes material items seem so small.

"Thanks, I appreciate you telling me all this. It's really helpful," I told her, unsure of whether or not *helpful* was really the right word to use. Was it really *helpful?* Or was it still *terrifying?*

"Anyway, I was wondering if we could maybe have an angel wing. Dad doesn't have any at home, and he said he really liked using them here, and . . ." I tried to think of more reasons, but the nurse cut me off.

"Oh, my gosh, of course!" she exclaimed. "I'll be right back."

She disappeared into the nurses closet and returned a few moments later, carrying a grocery bag full of angel wings, along with fitted sheets and top sheets for Mom's hospital bed. She walked around to meet me at my side, making it feel like some kind of drug deal. "Shh. Don't tell anyone," she whispered as she handed me the bag.

I peeked inside, glancing at all the linens she was providing to us, free of charge, and thanked her profusely.

"Thank you. Thank you for everything," I said earnestly. "Thank you for caring about Mom and my family so much. We were so lucky to have you as our nurse."

She pulled me into a hug and said, "You're welcome, sweetie. Let us know if there's anything else you need."

I nodded. "I will."

As I left the hospital that day, I was grateful for the angel wing. But I was even more grateful for that angel nurse.

*_*_*_*_*_*

A few weeks later, during one of my visits with Mom, I decided to try on her wedding gown. She had it in her head that we might be able to alter it so I could wear it on my wedding day.

As I slipped the gown on over my clothes, I couldn't help feeling less than impressed. Even Mom didn't seem to like the way the dress looked anymore. "I should have gotten it preserved," she admitted.

It was yellowed and wrinkled, and I wished that she had preserved it so it would still be ivory. It lacked that sense of beauty that new gowns had. Also, it was a few inches too short for me. The chest would need to be lowered, and I would want to cut the back out so I could have an open-back dress like I had always dreamed of. The sleeves would also need to come off to accommodate my dream of a V-neck. All in all, it might cost more money to alter the gown than it would to buy a new one. Still, if for whatever reason Mom couldn't make it to my wedding, I had a feeling I might end up getting it altered and wearing it anyway.

With her wedding dress still on me, I asked her what she wanted for her future.

"Do you think you'll make it to my wedding?" I asked her hopefully. "I mean, you were just admitted into hospice . . ." I felt like it wasn't something I should admit out loud to her, even though we both knew it was true.

"I don't want to live like this," she replied.

I understood that it wasn't that she didn't want to live. She just didn't want to live like *that*. In a bed. Unable to move. Unable to participate.

I didn't blame her. I really didn't. I just hoped she knew that when she felt like she was ready to quit, we would all understand and we would all be okay.

I took off the dress and pulled out her iPad. I sat next to her on her bed and together, we browsed through a website where she could order new glasses. She wanted a new pair for my wedding. *So maybe she did intend on going?* I was so confused.

She spent rest of the spring and into the summer trying to find a dress to wear to my wedding, which would be in October at a small inn in New Hampshire. She tried to coordinate a *chuppah* for the wedding ceremony. A *chuppah* was an important symbol in a Jewish wedding ceremony. It was a canopy that the couple stood under while taking their vows, and it was supposed to represent the home that they would build together. It was open on all four sides to represent the idea that friends and family would always be welcome there. She also tried to find a pretty aisle runner so my dress wouldn't get grass stains. If it didn't rain, we anticipated holding the ceremony outdoors in front of the pond.

Visiting with her was like looking through a kaleidoscope. Depending on which way you tilted the lens and how you turned the scope, you could get a variety of images. With Mom, it depended on the exact moment as to what you would receive. One moment we would be talking about wedding dresses, and the next moment her hand needed to be moved an inch, and she would cry in relief after we moved it. It was those tiny moments that brought me back to reality and reminded me that everything was really not okay. Like when we turned her feet outward to stretch them after they had been turned inward for hours and she cried. Or when we fixed the crinkled sheet behind her back, and it made all the difference in the world. Or when I hugged her good-bye, and she sobbed on my shoulder and her grief transferred through our touch. When she couldn't even lift her arms to hug me back, and she was so, so sad.

Sometimes, when it was just she and I, we talked honestly about how miserable she was. I'd wipe her face and tell her everything was okay. But when her friends were there, she put on a front like everything was fine and like she didn't totally hate her life. She was constantly putting on masks and taking them down.

She didn't want to live like this; she wanted to get better. Sometimes she cried for no real reason. Dad always asked why she was crying and tried to get her to stop. I would just hug her and rest my head lightly on her shoulder until she calmed herself down. I never thought she needed to stop. She had a right to be sad.

And then someone would come visit and temporarily distract us again. They would talk about their own drama and Mom would get opinionated and spirited again. She would be distracted for a while until something else hurt or until she tried to do something like lift her sippy cup and didn't have the strength.

Dad would put her in her wheelchair while he changed her sheets and fixed up the bed. She didn't like it though, because sitting crushed her stomach and caused her pain. I hoped maybe eventually it won't hurt so bad.

How's Your Mom?

Maybe, eventually, none of us would hurt as much anymore.

CHAPTER FORTY-FOUR

MICHELLE

In March 2016, three months after the night Mom almost died, my parents celebrated their thirty-second wedding anniversary.

Mom said thirty-two years went by really fast, but I felt like that was a really long time to hang out with the same person every day. Over the years, I'd watched their love transform and grow as life unfolded in front of them, not that it looked easy, effortless, or even enjoyable at times. I'm not going to pretend like their relationship was always this beautiful, magical fairytale romance filled with rainbows and butterflies. Truthfully, it was far from it. At least from my perspective.

When Alex and I were little kids, my parents used to yell a lot. Sometimes it was at us because we were acting like brats or "skating on thin ice," as Mom used to say. Sometimes my parents would yell at each other. Dad would tell Mom to "go to hell," and Mom would respond with "I'm already there!" As a kid hearing those words, I was terrified it meant they didn't love each other anymore. I used to think my parents would surely get a divorce. I remember Mom telling Dad that she would always choose us over him and that she if she left him, she would take us with her. Again, this was terrifying to hear, but it was also oddly comforting to know she would always put us first, even before her own marriage. She always put us first.

My perspective as a child was like seeing their relationship through a broken TV screen. I wasn't on the inside, so I never really saw the whole picture. I saw pieces and fragments of their story, and I definitely didn't pay attention to everything that was going on. My judgments and fears were formed from moments in time, snippets of their lives when I felt like having the TV on. I didn't see it all.

Maybe that's why it took me a few years to really understand their love, or to understand love in general, for that matter.

All those Disney movies teach us that one day your Prince Charming will land magically in your path, look into your eyes, and fall madly in love with you. You're always told that relationships will take hard work and compromise, but you're never really shown what that looks like in a realistic context. What does hard work mean in a marriage? What does it take to compromise? These aren't things you learn by watching Disney movies, that's for sure. The only way you really learn it is to see it or live it yourself, in real life.

I'd learned that love isn't about rainbows and smiles. It turns out that while being stubborn is overrated and not ideal, it's often preferable to swallowing your pride, which is a really difficult thing to do. My parents showed me how to put the other person's needs first, above your own, for the sake of the relationship and the sake of your love.

What does it mean to put their needs before your own? Well, for Dad, it meant giving up everything to take the best possible care of Mom. For Mom, it meant lying uncomfortably for long amounts of time in bed, waiting for Dad to check on her because she wanted to give him as much space as she still could.

More importantly, and maybe even most importantly, my parents showed me how to persevere when things get hard. How to remain committed to each other. How to stand by each other and support each other, even when you don't completely agree with the decision the other person is making. Or, when you don't have a choice over the decision they're making. When fate makes decisions for you, you have to learn how to adapt to them. Mom's diagnosis of MS became a "sink or swim" situation for their marriage and continuously tested their love every day. Yet somehow, every day, they passed the test with flying colors. They showed me that true love was real, but it didn't come free. Like everything else in life, a good relationship took hard work and dedication. But when you worked at it and committed to it, it was so, so sweet.

CHAPTER FORTY-FIVE

CHRIS

The hospital bills began stacking up immediately after we brought her home.

Thankfully, she'd made it through; but it also meant I couldn't use the money from her life insurance to pay anything off. I was lucky that I had been able to continue to work full-time at my own small business, which I ran from the basement of my home. Between my paychecks and Tammy's Social Security, we made enough money to pay the minimum amount on our bills. We barely scraped by paying the minimum on the hospital bills, too. But I couldn't stress about those when I was so worried about Tammy every day.

Neither one of us had health insurance. Hospice took care of Tammy's medications and care, and that didn't cost us anything. Every six weeks, Tammy was reevaluated for continued admittance in the hospice program. Every time, we would panic that they might kick her out. They could very well decide that she was getting better and force her out of the program. But they never did. Instead, they told us she was progressively getting worse, and that they wanted to continue making her comfortable.

The irony was that without the ostomy surgery, we would have never been eligible for hospice care. It took something horrible to allow us to receive the care Tammy needed.

If you ask me, that's a broken healthcare system.

How's Your Mom?

CHAPTER FORTY-SIX

MICHELLE

Five months after the surgery, Mom had a particularly bad day. As she lay in bed, barely responsive and in unbelievable pain and discomfort from constipation, sucking the water off of the tiny sponge that I held in her mouth, I had a strong sense of déjà vu: We had been here before.

In between squeaky phrases and gasps for air, she apologized for whining and continued to tell me she was nauseous and miserable. She whimpered about being thirsty but was unable to drink. I reminded her that when she'd been in the ICU for a week, her only source of liquid came off those tiny sponges on a stick. She was thirsty then, too, but she was okay. I told her that if anyone could face extreme thirst, it was her. She said "okay," and "I love you," and I hoped she believed me.

The tricky thing was that it wasn't normal constipation she was experiencing that day. She was constipated because her damn MS was taking the very last thing she had left: her digestive system. The nerves that instructed her digestive system to keep things flowing had stopped communicating with her brain. So she lay in bed, bloated, uncomfortable and miserable.

I stroked her face with a cool washcloth and rubbed her stomach where she said it hurt. Finally, the morphine kicked in, and she began to fall asleep. With her blankets pulled up to her chin, she looked comfortable and almost angelic.

As I watched her sleep, I was filled with flashbacks of the fear of losing her; of the look on Dad's face, so scared and crippled; of the text messages that circulated between all my family members with constant questions and updates. This was all too familiar.

I was still staring at Mom when my cell phone vibrated in my hand. My Auntie Trudy was calling me. She was a retired nurse and had the kindest, gentlest soul of anyone I had ever known. I loved my Auntie Trudy more than anyone else in the world, and she was my favorite person to talk to about Mom, even though

I didn't do it often. She had always told me I could call her, but I never did. Talking about it seemed pointless to me because it wouldn't make anything better.

I walked quickly through the living room and kitchen, then locked myself in the laundry room. Dad was around the house somewhere, and I didn't want him to hear my conversation. I scooted myself onto the washing machine, then took a deep breath, doing my best to collect myself for her. I slid my finger across the "answer" button.

"Hi!" I said, sounding and feeling genuinely happy to hear from her.

"Hi, Michelle," she said warmly. "How's it going?"

"Fine," I lied, the way I always did. "I'm at my parents' now."

"Oh, good!" she cheered. "How's your mom?"

"She's on a lot of drugs," I began. "She seems really sick. She told me that she thinks she's going to die full of shit. She wants us to write that on her tombstone: *Died the same way she lived: Full of shit.*"

She laughed, so I did, too. Then she exhaled deeply, allowing the reality of the situation to sink in.

"Do you really think this is the end?" she asked after a few quiet moments.

I was shocked by her question, even though I knew I shouldn't be. "I don't know," I told her honestly. "On the one hand, it's just constipation, right?"

"Right," she replied.

"Obviously no one has ever died from that before," I continued. "So maybe the drugs will kick in soon, and everything will start working again. Maybe this will all be no big deal."

I continued without letting Auntie Trudy speak. "On the other hand, it's technically a complication of MS, and people do die from those. Even if she takes drugs for constipation, they won't fix her broken nerves."

"Oh, Michelle . . ." Auntie Trudy cooed. I could tell that she didn't know what to say; she didn't have any answers. I suddenly felt bad for being so honest with her. That was why I hated telling the truth—it made people sad.

"How are you doing?" she asked.

"I'm just confused. We have no idea what might happen," I admitted, my teeth beginning to chatter. "She might all of a sudden start pooping, and everything could go back to normal. Or she could die tonight!"

I couldn't believe I'd said it out loud. The words had just fallen out of my mouth. *She could actually die tonight*, I thought to myself. The possibility suddenly felt tangible.

"It's okay to accept what you're really feeling," Trudy encouraged. I felt a tear fall from my face and watched it splash aggressively on my jeans. It left a giant wet circle. I tried to wipe it dry with the palm of my hand, but I couldn't. I just smeared the moisture around and made the circle bigger. I remained silent, staring at the temporary stain on my jeans. I didn't know what I was really feeling. I was hoping she would tell me.

"We're afraid of her getting better, not of her dying, aren't we?" she finally asked, then caught her breath. She was crying, too. *Yes*, I realized. *That was what I was feeling. How did she know?*

"If she gets better, she's just going to have to face something else." I practically screamed it, shoving the tears off the sides of my face, too angry to let any more fall. "If she *gets better*, she's still going to have MS!"

My whole body was shaking. Auntie Trudy sniffled.

"She will just go back to living a life that *isn't even living*," I said, my voice completely consumed with attitude. I sounded like I was thirteen. *Who WAS I? Why did I sound like I wanted my mom to die?*

"I know," Auntie Trudy said. "It's all going to be okay. We will all get through this together."

"I know," I repeated back to her. For a few moments, neither of us spoke. We just let each other cry.

"I'm glad you called," I eventually told her. "I'm really glad I have you, and I love you," I said. *Family is everything*, I realized suddenly.

"I love you too, sweetie," she said. "Call me if you need anything, okay?"

"I will," I promised, thinking that maybe I actually would this time.

After we hung up, I couldn't help but acknowledge the thoughts that were screaming at me in my mind. Mom was my best friend. I didn't want to lose her under any circumstances. But I did want her to find peace. I had no idea what would happen or how I would react when it did. All I knew is that G-d really did have a plan for all of us, and everything happened for a reason. I had to believe that everything would work out the way it was supposed to. It was the only way I would be able to fall asleep that night.

˷˷*˷*˷*˷*

Over the course of the next few days, her health continued to decline. The stool softeners, laxatives, nerve stimulators, muscle relaxers, stomach coaters, and everything else we pumped into her system seemed to have no effect on her ability to move waste through her digestive system. Her stomach continued to grow. She woke in pain in the middle of the night when her medicines wore off. She hallucinated and needed Dad to turn on the lights to make them stop. She saw her mother in her sleep.

During the day, she told us all kinds of "Tammyisms" that only made partial sense. Maybe it was the morphine. She explained how the Jewish tradition believed that the soul shatters into tiny pieces when someone dies and that the living will see sparks of the deceased's soul wherever they are. She told me that her sparks would be all around me. I believed in this because I remembered feeling those sparks everywhere I went when I thought she was going to die the last time.

She flip-flopped between wanting to die and wanting to stay alive. She told me I was a "good girl," and apologized profusely. She told me I would be all right, and that she was glad I had Tyler. She was sorry she wouldn't make it to our wedding.

She asked for things like hot lemon water, hot lattes, and cranberry juice, and took small sips to stay as hydrated as possible. She took tiny tastes of applesauce, but she hadn't eaten a real meal for six days. There was nowhere for the food to go.

She was on steroids and painkillers that altered her personality significantly. She said things that I knew she didn't mean and she didn't really look at me when I was talking. Sometimes she said things that sounded like Mom, but most of the time, I could barely recognize her speaking.

"I want there to be peanut butter and jelly sandwiches at my funeral," she told me once. "And chocolate milk." I actually wrote it down, certain that when she died, I would forget her requests.

"Make sure you look for me in the sparks surrounding you," she reminded me. "And make sure you tell people that I died full of shit." She laughed to herself before falling asleep again.

˷˷*˷*˷*

Magically, a few days later, her digestive system started working again. And all of our lives, somehow, carried on.

CHAPTER FORTY-SEVEN
CHRIS

There were so many times that year that I thought she was a goner. She came right to the precipice of dying too many times. Morphine gave her nightmares, so the hospice nurses put her on a liquid drug called Dilaudid. We called it "purple haze" because it did seem to put her in a hazy, happy state. It was supposedly stronger and better than morphine. I gave her huge doses of it, and each time, I thought to myself, *She is a goner. This is where she is going to die.* I said my good-byes every time she fell asleep.

But she didn't die. The ailment always passed. She always stayed.

One night, she said she had been visited by an angel. "It looked like Michelle," she told Alex, Michelle, and me the following day. "She wore a pink t-shirt, and her curly blonde hair was tied back in a ponytail. She came and sat on the end of my bed." She pointed to the place where the angel had sat. "She just watched me for a while, and then she left because she was done. I guess it wasn't my time to go home yet."

People always wanted to know how she was doing. I had to tell them I didn't know how long she would last. One day she was good, and the next day she wanted to check out.

Nobody could predict the future.

CHAPTER FORTY-EIGHT

MICHELLE

On a warm, sunny day in October 2016, I stood in front of all of my family and friends, preparing to recite my vows to the very best friend I had ever had. It was a perfect fall day in New Hampshire as Tyler and I stood in front of a gorgeous pond, which effortlessly reflected the foliage of the trees surrounding it. We were holding hands, *finally* getting married. Mom and Dad sat side by side in the front row. Dad's right arm was casually wrapped around Mom's shoulders, reminding me of two teenagers on a first date. As I looked at them, Dad used his free hand to wave to me. I smiled back.

Mom's friend, who had also been an optician at Nashua Eye Professionals, had spent the morning getting her ready, doing everything from putting on her pantyhose to applying her mascara and curling her hair. Dad wore the gray suit that matched the ones Tyler's groomsmen were wearing, accompanied by a solid black tie. I had to admit, he cleaned up pretty well. But no one at our wedding looked as good as Mom.

I thought back to the first six months of the year when I'd been so worried about whether or not she was going to die, how I wanted to soak up every possible moment with her and how I visited her every chance I got. I even took days off from work just to be with her. I made sure to talk to her every day, even if it was just a simple text. I always said "I love you" when I left.

In July, when she finally picked out a dress for my wedding, I hoped that meant things were settling down enough that I could trust she would make it to my wedding, but I could never be certain she would. Dad frequently reminded me, all year long, that there was a chance she might not live to make it.

Now, as I looked at her in the champagne-colored gown we had purchased together online, I felt another small victory inside of me. *She had beaten MS again.* The gown was adorned with sequins and sparkled all over. It was short-sleeved and floor-length, and it looked absolutely stunning on her. I smiled at my parents, then looked back at Tyler, and then to his parents in the front row on the opposite side of us. His mom, dad, and stepdad all looked amazing, too. I could practically feel the pride beaming off of each one of them. They felt like family to me, too, and I looked at them almost the same way I had looked at my own parents. *How had I gotten so lucky?*

Miraculously, I didn't cry at all while I recited my vows. But Tyler did while he read his, even though he wasn't a crier. I had only seen him cry once before, when he said his last good-byes to his grandfather. His tears had actually started when I met him at the end of the aisle. One dainty tear was falling down his left cheek, wrapping itself around his chin, and it made me smile. Then, he cried again while reading me his vows. I couldn't believe I didn't cry, especially when he did.

The truth was, while I was amazed and ecstatic to be marrying him, the act of doing so felt so natural and *right* that I wasn't even close to crying. Marrying him was just what I was supposed to do. It was almost matter-of-fact. I was the luckiest girl in the world, yes, and I couldn't believe how much I loved him, but it didn't make want to cry the way so many other things had during the past year. Maybe I just didn't know how to cry happy tears anymore.

I did cry later on, though, as Dad and I shared our father-daughter dance. Dad cried first, and he kept trying to wipe away his tears while we danced together. Neither one of us could believe that Mom was there to watch us. The whole year had been such a turbulent whirlwind of uncertainty. As we laughed through our tears, Dad said, "My siblings are never gonna let me live this down." Dad was the second youngest of seven, and all his siblings and my cousins were watching us intently. As macho and masculine as he was, there was something so sweet and touching about dancing with his baby girl. And to top it off, we were crying. We must have looked like a couple of idiots. I didn't care. I was so proud of my Dad after all we had been through.

As I wrapped my arms around Dad's neck, I caught a shimmering glimpse of my engagement ring, resting beautifully next

How's Your Mom?

to my brand new wedding band. They were *so* sparkly. Tyler had let me exchange my engagement ring a few weeks after he proposed. When we went to purchase wedding bands, I told him that I couldn't find a wedding band that matched the engagement band, which was true. The tiny twists made it so that neither straight or curved bands looked good next to it. I ended up purchasing a brand-new set of matching rings. Tyler felt horrible for "screwing everything up," but to me, he didn't screw anything up. The fact that I felt honest enough with him to tell him that I wanted to exchange it was all I cared about. Honesty was what mattered in a relationship.

Later on, after Tyler and I cut our cake, and my veil completely fell out of my hair, as the night was beginning to wind down, I heard a familiar song come over the DJ's speakers. I hadn't asked our DJ to play it. It wasn't really a popular song anymore and wasn't a normal song to play at weddings. I had never even heard it at a wedding before.

"I hope you never lose your sense of wonder . . ." I immediately handed Tyler the glass of white wine I had been sipping on and said, "I'll be right back. This is our song." He looked at me, confused. He might have thought I meant it was *our* (as in Tyler and I's) song, but it wasn't. It was Mom and I's. I strutted across the dance floor, holding my gown above my ankles, admiring my white sparkly Keds that Hannah had given to me as a gift the night before.

I found Mom at her table, where a few relatives had been sitting next to her, chatting. "I'm sorry," I rudely interrupted. "I need my mom." Without missing a beat, I switched on her electric wheelchair and brought it to the dance floor. I parked her in the middle of all of our family and friends, who were slow-dancing to it, and I said, *"Listen."*

Lee Ann Womack sang, *"I hope you dance . . ."* Mom's entire face lit up as her jaw hit the ground. I could practically see the lyrics floating magically across the entire ballroom. "It's our song!" she squealed excitedly.

I laughed, nodded my head, and then sat down on her lap,

dancing with her the only way I knew how. I rested my head on her right shoulder and listened as she sang the words to me along with Lee Ann. *"I hope you never fear those mountains in the distance . . . Never settle for the path of least resistance . . ."*

I watched her for a few moments. *"Livin' might mean takin' chances, but they're worth takin', Lovin' might be a mistake, but it's worth makin',"* she sang, then looked back at me before continuing. *"Give the heavens above more than just a passing glance . . ."*

"Mom?" I interrupted while lifting my head up from her shoulder.

"Shell?"

"I'm so glad you're here," I told her.

"Me, too."

Lee Ann kept continued singing. *"Promise me that you'll give faith a fighting chance . . . and when you get the choice to sit it out or dance . . ."* Just then, Hannah, Noreen, and Tyler joined us in the middle of the dance floor, as the music got quiet in preparation for the greatest crescendo of the song. They formed a circle around Mom and me, wrapped their arms around each other, and sang out loud with Mom and me. *"I hope you dance!"*

If there was one thing Mom taught me that I would always remember, it's that when you got the choice to sit it out or dance. . . . you should *dance*.

Always, always, dance.

*ˎ*ˎ*ˎ*ˎ*ˎ*

As the new year rolled around, and the anniversary of the night she almost died came and went, my family finally had a day where we got together for lunch, just the six of us. We had gotten so used to extended family members constantly visiting that we barely realized how much we all missed the intimacy of our immediate family.

For a short while, it was just like how things used to be before the surgery. We all happily ate steak and potatoes at the kitchen table, and Mom ate about five Girl Scout cookies. We laughed and told stories, just like we used to.

That night, I started to see, with some level of clarity, how lucky we had been to survive the past year and how much we could all learn from it.

If the past year had never happened, I would have never known what it would feel like to lose her, and I would have continued feeling sorry for myself and angry at her MS until it was too late.

Before last year, I thought I knew what it felt like to lose my mom. I really thought I did. I thought that when I looked at her, sitting in her living room chair, playing Words with Friends on her iPad all day, that I didn't know who she was. I thought MS had stolen all of the pieces of Mom that made her who she was. Before, when I looked at her, I didn't see her anymore. I saw a ghost of what she used to be, and only shreds of her remained. I thought she was already gone.

I thought I already knew what it felt like to lose her.

But I had no idea.

Before the incident with her shoulder, I *hated* everything she had *lost*. After the incident, I was *grateful* for everything she still *had left*. She could still help me with table arrangements for my wedding. She could still watch movies with me. She could still eat cake with me! She could still listen to my stories and give me advice. She was still only a phone call away. She was still the same mom she always was, and I was still so lucky to have her.

It was possible that, if the past year hadn't happened, I wouldn't have realized any of that.

CHAPTER FORTY-NINE

TAMMY

At the end of 2016, I didn't bother to do the year-end assessment like I usually did. I used to enjoy looking back on the year and seeing what I could or couldn't do. I liked reflecting on who I was and who I had become and dreaming about the type of person I would someday be. Of course, that was when I thought I would get better.

Now the end of the year assessment seemed kind of fruitless, as the MS was mixed in with the shoulder surgery recovery. The two just blended together. Was it due to the surgery that I spent more time in bed, or was it the MS progressing that forced me to become more bedridden?

After a year and a half, I thought I had recovered from the surgery. If I were a well person, I would have been back in the game. Even with the ostomy bag, I thought I could have been back to a new normal. But where did the MS leave me? I stayed in bed because it was easier for everyone. I was comfortable and safe, and I could entertain myself with the way I set up my iPad on my lap and my little table at my bedside.

I never thought my bedroom would get as much traffic as it did. I used to dream of having a master bedroom with a white carpet. Now, the white carpet had become the bane of Chris's existence, as all he saw were the spots on the rug. He constantly wanted to get out the carpet cleaner to clean it. As my neat and tidy little house fell to disarray all around me, I reassured Chris that he was doing the best he can. It was all those little womanly touches that left the house lacking.

I could only use my right hand, and that, too, was fading. It was useless by the end of the day. On the plus side, I discovered that using a stylus helped me do things on my iPad. So the diminishing use of my hand did not leave me frustrated and sad; instead, I was proud of myself for finding another new way to do things.

When I sat back and thought of life before MS, it was too

painful to remember. It became a futile exercise in chronological notations to think of life with MS before the wheelchair. Why remember when I was just walking with the cane? Or when I could transfer myself from toilet to my Jazzy Blue wheelchair? Or when I could drive my Jazzy Blue out onto the deck? At each stage of my disease, I wondered, at that time, what it would mean to get worse. I knew I was in denial thinking *it couldn't get any worse*. It always did.

Now, I simply felt grateful for what I knew was coming next but had not yet happened. I knew that eventually, I would lose what remained of my right hand. I knew that I would choke more and lose my ability to swallow. I knew I wouldn't be able to eat at all. I was grateful I could have hospice take care of me. They knew I did not want to be fed by a tube, or have nutrition pumped into me through an IV.

I thought about the treatments that had been available to those of us living with PPMS five years ago. Chronic Cerebrospinal Venous Insufficiency (CCVI) was a trial procedure of opening the vein that led to the brain from the spine in hopes that it would increase the blood flow and solve all the problems of MS. Although it was big news, I read about more failures than successes with that procedure, so I did not even pursue it in my thoughts.

Now, five years later, there was a buzz about stem cell research. This approach was proving to be more successful, and many patients with the relapsing types of MS felt it was a cure. Even people with PPMS were saying it halted the progression. Five years ago, this would have been a dream come true for me. But now, it was too late.

When I had chemotherapy, doctors dumped small amounts of Cytoxan into my veins to try to slow the progression. At the time, I was still walking with a cane or a walker, and I still could get myself washed up or have Chris put me in the shower. I could still get dressed, sometimes with help and sometimes alone. I could still wear pants, and I could make it to the bathroom in time (most times). Oh, if I could only have stopped the progression back then.

That was what the stem cell treatment was doing now.

When I was undergoing chemo, I was probably a four on the disability scale, which ranges from zero to ten. Now I was an eight or nine. It made no sense to try to stop the progression at this point. All that meant was that I'd spend my life lying in bed with someone constantly caring for me. At this stage, I was a burden for all of those around me who cared for me and loved me.

Stem cell treatments were generating hope. It was being done in some other countries, but not here in the United States. It was still at the trial stages here. People were traveling across the globe in search of treatments. And some were finding ways to prolong their lives.

I told my family right from the beginning, I was not the type of person who would go globe-trotting searching for a cure. Even if I did decide to pursue it, at that point in my progression, the only place that would accept me as a patient was Israel. And it would cost so much money—$150,000 for the procedure, which did not include transportation and accommodations for the person who would have to travel with me. Not to mention how difficult it was for me to travel. It made me angry that this procedure was not being done here in the United States due to lack of FDA approval.

On the one hand, we are all grateful for the FDA's efforts to keep us safe. On the other hand, people who were as desperate as I was to find some hope, even just a glimmer, did not have the option to pursue this kind of treatment in the US.

CHAPTER FIFTY

MICHELLE

It was another Thursday afternoon in my parents' bedroom. I had gotten in the habit of stopping by their house after work. After a few minutes of small talk and playing with the dog, Mom decided to get real again by telling me that she didn't want to live like this. I had heard her say things to that effect way too many times, so it was beginning to feel normal. It took me a moment to allow myself to be drawn into her thoughts.

"It's like whatever is hiding behind the curtain won't even show its ugly head," she told me.

"What do you mean?" I asked, although I was pretty sure she meant that she wished MS would just kill her already.

"It's like I can't even fight it," she continued.

"I feel like you have fought it, and you won," I countered.

"I can't do anything without someone else. Anything I do involves someone else's help. Even if someone comes over to visit, I have to ask for help. Dad says I don't have to ask . . . but of course I do. I have to make sure that someone can open and close the door, and they can come in, and that there's a chair for them to sit in, and offer them something to eat . . ." She paused, thinking of all the little ways most people cater to their house guests without even realizing it.

"People don't come over here because they want something to eat," I said, laughing.

"What if they want a cookie and a cup of tea?" she joked in return.

"I know what you mean, though, because I remember when you used to fight so hard to maintain your independence," I told her.

"I had to get up and take a shower every day!" She laughed as her eyes met mine.

I nodded. "I remember that."

"It was short lived, but I tried so hard to do that. I used to think you had to get showered and dressed every day. But I can't anymore."

Moments of silence ticked by before she attempted to change the subject. "Are you going to your cousin's birthday party next week? I get the impression she is having various birthday parties . . . one for the family and one for the kids . . . maybe you'll find out."

"That's good," I replied, completely uninterested in discussing my cousin's birthday party, wanting to stay on the current topic.

When I didn't take her bait, she tried switching to another topic. "What show should I watch when I finish binge-watching *Parenthood*?" She thought for a moment. "Maybe I'll re-watch the first season of *This is Us*."

She was good. She knew how much I loved *This is Us* and *Parenthood*. Bringing up two of my favorite TV shows made it *almost* impossible for me to ignore her sidetracked conversation. But I did.

"Who can you talk to? Who understands the frustration you must be feeling?" I asked her. *The Wheelchair Kamikaze* blog flashed in my head. She had reached out to the blog's author many times in the past. He always replied with very helpful, comforting information. "Maybe you could write Marc another email?"

"Maybe I'll send him another email. But it's like we said, even if the Phase Two stem cell trial at the Tisch Center in NYC starts in June, how long will it take before they have results? How long will it take for them to talk about them and start offering treatment?" She sighed. "I was thinking about writing something on the MS Society's Connection page. But every time I look at it, it's just people who are looking for sympathy."

"Are there other people who are in your shoes?" I wondered out loud, thinking there was often comfort in numbers, to know that you weren't the only one going through something. "I just want to know what other people do. The way you're living right now is just so . . . *screwed up.*" It was harsh, but I knew she wouldn't mind if I spoke honestly. "I've never known anyone else that has lived the way you have for so long."

"That is homebound . . ." she added.

"Yeah! And in hospice care."

"I got lucky," she replied. As if on cue, our dog, Lucky, perked his ears in excitement. Lucky had previously belonged to Tyler and me, but he couldn't be left alone because he had terrible separation anxiety. He was much happier living with Honeybee and my parents, who were home all day. Lucky leapt to his feet and began wagging his tail as he trotted over toward the chair where I was sitting, next to my mother's hospital bed.

"Not Lucky the dog," she laughed. I joined her, this time grateful for a pause in the conversation.

A moment later, she lifted her right arm, which was barely working anymore, and attempted to readjust her glasses. She got them off her face and then tried to put them back on, but her arm didn't have enough strength to reach. Instead, she poked herself in the eye with them.

Again, she laughed, and I did, too. "I was trying to tuck them under my hair!"

I stood to help her, and then she continued our previous conversation.

"The MS Society tries to support people," she said.

"I know . . . but what support do we really need?" I asked curiously.

"Well, the last time my hospice nurse practitioner came to recertify me for hospice, she told me I would always have hospice because I have a progressive disease and it's progressively getting worse."

"So they're never going to cut you off or let you go because you're never going to get better," I spat without thinking. I hated my tendency to paint things in black and white. But sometimes, that's how I saw them. "Super!" I scoffed, knowing I sounding like a hormonal, sarcastic teenager, and loathing myself for it.

"Right."

"Well, it makes you wonder if maybe you should voluntarily leave the hospice program to try to find treatment, and if you can't, then . . ."

"That would mean that Dad would have to bring me to all kinds of doctors, and what good would that do? Plus, I already did that," she reminded me. "We have to remember that I did that when I was trying to get diagnosed. I was going to a different doctor every single week. I would go on my lunch hour or get out of work early. You gotta remember that."

"Yeah, I do," I said softly.

"I had all those back surgeries, hoping it was my back . . . remember that? Now that's all I think about. I'm getting so self-centered. I'm sure you have many more stories to tell than I do, but I just lay here and think about myself." Tears began forming in the front of her eyes again.

"I would, too, if I were you. I don't blame you."

"I don't like being this way, though. I like hearing other people's stories."

Even if I did have a happy story to share, I wouldn't have shared it because I didn't want to change the subject. I was too grateful to be speaking openly, honestly, the way we used to in our book. I needed more information, more honesty.

"What do you really want?" I asked, hoping it didn't sound too snarky.

"I want to be cured," she replied, with a struggle in her voice. "I don't want MS anymore. That's what I want."

I already knew this, and the truth was, it wasn't the answer I was hoping for. I wanted her to say something actionable. Something we could have control over. "What do you want that's realistic?" I asked, again, sounding like a bitchy thirteen-year-old, even as I smiled to try to soften the blow. I wasn't trying to be a bitch. I was just trying to be honest.

Seconds ticked by. She didn't have an answer.

I backpedaled, feeling instantly terrible for implying that she might really *never* get better. Even if it was true, it was not the kind of thing you were supposed to say out loud. "If you wait for stem cell therapy, it would stop you from getting worse. But would it bring you back to what you used to be?"

　　　　　　　　　　　　　　　　　　How's Your Mom?

"Well, that's what they're trying to see. Maybe there will be nerve regeneration to reverse it."

I stared at her, wishing I had all the answers, wishing I knew exactly what the future held for stem cell therapy. Again, I assumed the role of caregiver, of nurturer and supporter, feeling less like a daughter and more like a mom. It was the way things had been since she had gotten diagnosed. I wanted so badly to fix her broken world, the way a mom would bandage her toddler's skinned knee.

"It's not gonna happen in my lifetime," she said, finally giving me something black and white that I could understand. Her facade cracked again. Her face was like a glass window that had been pressed on too hard. Tears spilled down her cheeks as my own began to fall. Her pain was contagious. "I wish I had cancer," she whispered, wiping her nose with a tissue.

It might have sounded insensitive to someone who didn't know her. But to me, it didn't. Instead, it spoke volumes about how she felt, about how difficult it was to live with MS. It was so hard that you would literally rather have cancer, because at least then you'd have the chance of an expiration date for your misery. I got it. I really did.

She paused, the silence forming a warm glow around us. Sometimes there were no words to fill the silence.

"It's so silly . . . Kristina is going to open a school," she continued, reverting back to her obsession with *Parenthood*. Kristina was a character, about Mom's age, on the show. "She beat cancer, now what is she going to do with her free time? Open a school!" she said, mockingly. "It's cute," she decided, while I pondered the notion that Mom would never have the chance to get better and open a school, or do anything she really cared about, for that matter. "It makes for a good story to watch," she concluded.

I ignored her third attempt to change the conversation and brought her back to reality. "That's what I'm so torn between. People who have cancer have the chance to fight it, or they die. I really don't know what's worse. I don't know whether I'm jealous of the kids who lose their parents quickly to cancer because they don't have to watch them suffer . . . or if I feel bad for them because they only get the limited time that they got."

She nodded, completely understanding, and not at all offended by my totally honest confession. I needed to get it off my chest.

"I know it's such a horrible thing to say," I admitted as I tucked a loose strand of hair behind my ear, unable to even meet her gaze. I could feel her looking at me, encouraging me to continue, silently letting me know that it was okay to feel that way.

"It's one of those questions . . . what would you rather be, blind or deaf?" she replied.

"Yeah. I'm grateful for all the extra time I got to spend with you, but I also hate seeing you like this."

"Right."

"You're not living!" I stammered, angry, shaking. The words poured out before I could stop them. I wondered, again, if my honesty crossed a line.

But I knew she understood when she responded with, "I'm existing."

I half-smiled back at her, grateful that she understood, but sad that we'd agreed on something so tragic.

"It's like I told you before. It's enough already," she said.

"If you had something you could do to try to get better, it would be a completely different story," I offered.

"Exactly! That's what I mean! If they told me *oh, just do this physical therapy and you'll get better,* and I had something to work at . . ." she paused.

"Yeah. It just sucks that it feels like you have no options."

She thought for a moment, then said, "I don't know of any options." She paused again. I racked my brain, searching for an answer, a glimmer of hope, anything to make her feel better. I had nothing. "It's just so unfair," she croaked, more tears spilling onto her nightgown.

"I know." I sighed, my heart aching more than I knew it could. We sniffled in unison.

"What if there really is reincarnation?" she asked me. Her

face was still so twisted, I couldn't tell if she was kidding or not. Was she trying to smile? She made a sort of hiccupping sound, and I couldn't figure out if it was a laugh or a small wail. "What if I come back in a shitty family?"

"Oh, is that what you're worried about?" I asked, unable to control my laughter.

She shook her head and replied, "No, I'm laughing!" She caught her breath. "Wouldn't that be horrible? Or maybe I'll come back as a dog. Wouldn't that be funny? People believe in reincarnation. I don't really know what I believe."

"Me, either."

"My mother always said 'I won't haunt you.'" I laughed as she continued, making the same promise to me. "I won't haunt you."

"You better not," I replied, again, only partially kidding.

"I won't." She paused again. "If it's possible . . ." She took a deep breath, seemingly gathering herself as I looked at her, soaking up every minute that she was still here with me, knowing I would miss these types of moments so much when she was gone. "If it's true that you can be there for certain things . . . then I'll be there." Her lower lip quivered as she dabbed tears from the corner of her eyes. I clung to the words, hoping with every fiber of my being, and wishing with all I had, that it would be true.

CHAPTER FIFTY-ONE

TAMMY

Some days I couldn't keep myself from falling into the pit of self-pity. I felt myself falling into that place, where no amount of distraction could keep me from falling. The tears came first, and the wrenching sobbing followed. I hated the sound of my crying. I didn't have a soft and pretty sounding sob. It wasn't quite a wail . . . it was more like the sound of a pig in pain. My nose ran, and that was not a lovely sight. I looked like a mess and sounded a mess. While wallowing in this pool, I found myself not so much counting the *used to be's*. I was not making a list of the things that I missed. That was the old school of self-pity. I had outgrown that and graduated to a new level beyond the *used to be's* to a level of realizing what would *never be*.

Most of it resulted from watching TV advertisements. The advertising and marketing experts had a way of making you want things. For me, it was the realization that I would never again need to acquire these things. I would never again get a new car. I would never go to Payless and get a new pair of shoes. I would never go to Kohl's or JCPenney to buy a new outfit. I would never need to buy new makeup. I would never go on a cruise or buy new furniture. I would never paint the walls in my house or buy new knickknacks to scatter among my stuff. I would never buy new curtains, sheets, carpets, towels, dishes or appliances. I would never cook or bake or use a Swiffer or Bounty paper towels to clean up everyday messes. I would never take a run through the woods. It hurt to think about how I would never play games with my grandchildren. I was living a life in limbo.

As I looked at the characters on the TV shows that I watched, I thought about how I would never again feel like the beautiful wife. I would always be on the outside looking in, a fly on the wall who saw all.

Sometimes it was nice to be a fly on the wall. I could almost see what life would be like when I was gone. Chris and Michelle would have nice chats in the kitchen, and Chris and Alex would play with their "man toys" in the basement. Life would go on.

I often wondered, *why was I still here?* I've asked a few people that question on the MS forums and one responder said it was because I still had hope. It got me to thinking, *just what exactly is hope?* I asked a friend, and she said, "You hope you are living this life that you are given in a good way." I tried to be gracious and thankful for those people who were around me, who helped me every day. I tried not to complain or be demanding. So, for that, I was hopeful that I could continue to be relatively cheery.

Another friend answered the question of hope as it pertained to being optimistic. "You hope everything goes well along the way. Even if the situation seems to be futile and the results unsure, you can only hope that you will see some bright spots in it all and that everything will work out in the end. Like, if you're running late for an appointment, you are hopeful that you won't get stuck in traffic, and that it will all work out in the end. You hope that you aren't late for the appointment."

And then, of course, there was the kind of hope where you just hope you leave the world a better place just by having been in it. You hope you have taught your children well, and they will remember everything you taught them.

CHAPTER FIFTY-TWO
MICHELLE

It was fourteen months after the surgery, seven years after the original diagnosis when she first brought it up. I shouldn't have been surprised, really. I should have known it was coming.

Maybe I didn't see it because I was hiding too frequently in my place of denial. Maybe if I had bothered to poke my head out every once in a while, I wouldn't have been so taken aback when she told me.

She brought it up so casually that I couldn't help but wonder if she thought I saw it coming. I wondered, *had she spent weeks dreading talking to me about it? Or did she tell me the first chance she got? Did she think I was expecting it?*

If I were in her shoes, would I have had the courage to tell my daughter what she told me?

The conversation started out like many others we had been having for the past year. She told me how much she hated living with MS, and how sorry she felt for Dad. She kept emphasizing that none of it was fair to him. "Poor Dad. He's sick of this. He didn't sign up for this," she reminded me for the millionth time. She told me how she didn't think she was going to get any better, how the stem cell research trials wouldn't accept her because she was already *too far gone.*

That's when she told me about the handful of pills she had been stashing in her bedside drawer.

About the conversation she'd had with her hospice nurse, whose job it was to make her comfortable, even if that didn't mean keeping her alive.

About how she had already discussed it with Dad.

Maybe I was so blindsided because it was the first time in months that I felt like she *wasn't* dying from something. Throughout the past year, things had kept trying to kill her. Her digestive system had shut down. A bedsore became infected. She'd had horrible reactions to new medicines. She choked every now and then.

It had been a while since something had tried to take her from us. It seemed as if her window for passing was, for the moment, closed. Like there wasn't any way she would die soon.

"I have to talk to you," she said. "Dad told me that. . . ." She paused as tears flooded her eyes. She seemed unable to catch her breath. She gasped at the air, and I wondered if she was choking. Her jaw made awkward up and down motions like she was chewing on the air. *What was wrong?*

She finally caught her breath. " . . . I had to . . ."

She paused, and I clung to her words. *Had to what?*

". . . . I had to . . ." she tried again, as tears skidded down her cheek.

I stared at her, each fragment dragging on for an eternity. *Why was she crying?*

" . . . say good-bye . . ."

Good-bye?

". . . . to you and Alex first."

The tears soaked her blanket. She hiccupped. She struggled, again, to catch her breath. She blinked hard and wiped her nose with a tissue, waiting for me to respond.

Since she'd been diagnosed, I tried never to let her see me cry. I always tried to be so strong whenever I was in front of her. I usually made sure I walked away before I lost it completely if only to spare her from witnessing the pain she caused me. But this time, I couldn't pretend. I looked directly into her eyes and let her see me cry. There weren't any words I could offer. Showing her my tears was all I could manage.

"I get it," I finally gulped. And we both sat there, crying.

After a few minutes, Dad walked into the room, curious as to what all the crying was about. He sat down with us and joined in our misery. After a few minutes of the three of us crying in unison, I began brainstorming all the ways we could fix things.

"What if we get a wheelchair van so we could take her out more?" I asked, feeling hopeful. "Or what if we hired a full-time nurse so Dad could have more freedom?"

Patiently, Dad explained how neither of those options was

feasible. Mom couldn't go out anymore; it was too hard for her. She couldn't hold her own head up. Hiring a full-time nurse wouldn't be that different from the three-times-a-week visits we already had from the hospice nurses.

I tried to think of more things we could do, but I could tell that shooting down every one of my ideas was destroying Dad. I knew he wished one of my ideas would make everything better . . . but he knew it wouldn't.

You would think, after the seven years Mom had been living with MS, I might have gotten used to the sight of Dad crying, but it never got easier.

As the tears began falling from his face, I knew I needed to stop pretending. Stop denying, stop wishing, stop hoping . . . and start accepting. Start *really* accepting. Not just the diagnosis. But the *impact* of the diagnosis on the rest of our lives. When she was first diagnosed, those pamphlets told me she wouldn't die. She wasn't supposed to die from this. But she was going to.

I didn't know if I was *supposed* to understand where she was coming from. Was I supposed to tell her that she was crazy? That she shouldn't do it? That I needed her to stay? That we would fix her? That we would somehow magically make everything all better if only she would continue to keep fighting? I knew, if I told her those things, I'd be lying. And I knew saying those things would show her I didn't understand what she was feeling.

And the thing was, I did understand. I really did.

If I was perfectly honest, I was actually really proud of her for what she was thinking about doing.

Ever since she'd been diagnosed, MS had dictated the things she'd been able and not able to do. She wanted to keep running? *Too bad.* She wanted to continue doing housework? *Nope, not happening.* She wanted to take her dogs for a walk around the block? *Absolutely not.* Okay, fine, but just let her make it to the bathroom on time. *HA! Stupid human. You will have no control over when and where you do your business.*

For years, her MS was a constant, overbearing villain who dictated her every move. It strangled her in every possible way. Although she did her best to "fight" it, MS had beaten her at so many of her own games.

Until today. Today, she *finally* had won the war. She wasn't just *stronger* than MS. She took MS by the collar, shook her fist in its face, and finally, after all these years, told it to *go fuck off*. MS was through with calling the shots. It was her turn again.

The fact that she felt empowered enough to do that made me pretty damn proud to be her daughter.

*_*_*_*_*_*

When a month had passed, I was still proud of her. I still thought she would do it.

When two months had passed, I was curious as to why she hadn't done it yet.

When three months had passed, I was confused as to why she hadn't done it yet.

When four months had passed, I asked her blatantly why she hadn't done it yet. She couldn't give me an answer.

When five months had passed, I began to let it go.

And when six months had passed, just as my sense of understanding, empathy, and acceptance was beginning to morph back into anger at her disease, I remembered her favorite phrase: *When man plans, G-d laughs.*

It meant that even though we, as humans, liked to think we had control over the course of our lives, we didn't. G-d was the only one with a plan.

I really thought she would take the pills. I thought she *wanted* to check out. I thought she was done. I thought that being "done" meant she was strong—that she had beaten MS—that she had won. I was so proud of her.

So why was she still here? Why didn't she give up? She had the means to. She knew we would understand. She knew we would still love her. Why did she continue to lie in bed each day? Why didn't she take the pills?

Maybe she didn't realize how much work she was to care for. Maybe she couldn't see how desperately we all needed to grieve for all that we had lost. What about everything she had said? Did she not realize how much pain we were keeping bottled inside us? Did she not realize how badly it hurt us to see her so sick every single day? Why did she insist on continuing on? What, exactly, was she holding out for?

Faith. That's what she was holding out for. That's what she was still hoping for. She was hoping G-d would do what he felt was right at the moment he felt it was right. She knew it wasn't up to her to make those kinds of decisions. It was up to G-d. You had to trust that when things seemed to be absolutely unbearable and falling apart, G-d would know when to step in and take over.

Even though we, as humans, like to pretend we're in control, that we hold all the power in our lives, sometimes, the truth is that we just *don't.* There are some calls, some decisions, that simply aren't ours to make. Even when it feels like the decision would be easy, like the answer is dangling on a limb hanging directly in front of you, it's not your place to grab it. It was your job to keep believing things would work out the way they were supposed to, and that even if you felt completely alone, you weren't.

No, she wouldn't ever take the pills. She would only put her trust in G-d. It didn't matter how long it took. He would do it when the time was right.

CHAPTER FIFTY-THREE

ALEX

"How will we know when she's going to die?" Michelle asked me one Thursday afternoon.

We were in our parent's bedroom, visiting our Mom, who had voluntarily chosen to stop eating about a month ago. She had decided that she didn't want to die by chocking. She decided she was done letting MS control her. She didn't want a feeding tube. Who could blame her?

I continued to stop by religiously every day to see her after work, just like I had been doing for the past twenty months. During the first couple of days when she wasn't eating, I still offered her some of her favorite things—chocolate, graham crackers, and cookies. I knew she was serious about not eating when she wouldn't even take a piece of chocolate. I knew this was the beginning of the end.

Michelle wasn't always there at the same time I was, but this morning, I sent her a text message her to find out what time she would be there. Today, I wanted to be there with her. Today marked thirty days with very little water and no food. Mom hadn't been responsive for about a week. All she could do was breathe and sleep.

"She'll start mottling," I said, not looking her in the eye. I held my iPhone in between my hands horizontally, playing a game that I couldn't actually care less about. It was a stupid game. The graphics weren't even any good. I didn't know why I even bothered playing it.

"What's that?" she asked.

"It means her blood pressure starts to drop so her feet and hands will start to turn blue. They'll start feeling cold." I said, my gaze fixed completely on my phone screen. I'd been explaining things to her my entire life. To me, this was no different than explaining to her the difference in Internet speeds.

From the corner of my eye, I watched her stand from the

chair where she had been sitting at the end of Mom's bed. She peeled back the fleece blanket that was covering Mom's feet and pressed her hand to Mom's foot.

"It's cold," she said.

I looked up, caught her eye, and immediately looked away. I stood and took a step toward Mom, examining her legs.

"Yeah, see how her feet are getting blue? That means it's close," I said, pointing to the blotches of blue and purple that laid all over her calves and shins. My phone, still in my right hand, had dropped to my side during this revelation. Immediately after realizing this, I brought it back in front of my face and sat back down.

"Her feet are always blue," Michelle countered. "She has MS, you know."

"Yep. But this is different," I said.

I couldn't force myself to meet her eye again, but I knew my words must have stung. A second later, sure enough, she started sniffling. Oops. I didn't mean to make her cry. When she was an infant, and I was three years old, and I used her hair as a means to swing her back and forth in her baby swing . . . then, I might have been trying to make her cry. But now, I honestly didn't mean to.

"So . . . do you think she's, like, going to die tonight?" Michelle asked again, wiping a tear away.

Jesus, I couldn't help thinking. *How was I supposed to know?*

"Yeah, maybe," I said evenly. "Or tomorrow. I don't know. Soon."

"Oh," Michelle sighed again, then stood to take a piece of toilet paper from Mom's bedside table. Mom didn't buy tissues. It was one of her weird money-saving tricks.

It was possible that there was a tear in my eye, too, but I wouldn't let Michelle see it. I closed out of that stupid game and opened up a different one.

We sat in silence together for a while. Silence never bothered me. Didn't matter to me if I was in a room with someone and we weren't making small talk. Small talk was overrated.

Last Man Standing was playing on the TV behind Michelle's head, but it was on mute. Mom used to ask me to program

How's Your Mom?

her cable box every night because she didn't have the strength to change the channel herself. She would watch *Last Man Standing* from 6:00-7:00, *Wheel of Fortune* at 7:00, *Jeopardy!* at 7:30, and *Chronicle* at 8:00. For the last week, she hadn't been able to ask me to program them. But I did it anyway. I already knew the schedule, plus it was a habit of mine now.

Sometimes it seemed like I couldn't do much to help Mom. She was always Michelle's best friend. Michelle was always the one Dad asked to babysit her. My parents knew they could ask me for help if they needed it, but they always asked Michelle first. Mom and I were close, but we just didn't have as much in common as she and Michelle did. But she was my Mom and a damn good one at that. She put Michelle and me above everything else in her life. I knew how lucky I was to have her. Even if I didn't show it all the time, or tell her I loved her enough, she knew how much I appreciated her. She knew I'd never forget her. I know she knew I loved her. That was really all that mattered.

"Hey, what are you guys doing?" Dad asked us, walking into the room, wearing his clunky, dirty, ratty boots. Why did he need to wear his Timberland boots in August? His shirt had stains all over it. He was such a mess. I shook my head at him while he entered.

"Nothing," Michelle said.

"Shit!" I whispered, slapping my knee. I died and had to start my level over.

"What?" Dad asked.

"Nothing," I said, putting both hands back on my phone. Silence filled the room again.

"It's close, you guys," Dad breathed.

"Yep, we know," I stated, nonchalantly.

He walked to Mom's side and whispered in her ear. "How are you, baby?" He kissed her. Michelle took out her phone and started scrolling aimlessly with her thumb. Dad stood there, tucking Mom's hair behind her ear, then re-applied her Chapstick for the hundredth time. "Mmm . . . Chapstick," he said, licking his own lips while he put on an excessive amount.

Dad stood with us until Michelle's stomach started to growl, fifteen minutes later.

"I'm gonna go," she said.

"Yep. Me too," I echoed, then stood right up.

"Okay, guys. Drive safe. Don't be surprised if you get a phone call from me tonight," Dad said.

He shook my hand, then pulled Michelle in for a hug. "I love you," he told us, then boomed, "Go give your mother a kiss." Michelle walked to her first, placed her head on Mom's chest for a few seconds, kissed her on the forehead and said, "I love you."

I approached her next, giving her a quick peck on the cheek and said, "Love you, Mom."

Then Michelle, Dad, and I walked together toward the exit of the bedroom. I took one last look at Mom, lying there so peacefully like she had for almost two whole years. G-d, she had had enough. She was done. She was so done. I couldn't blame her one bit.

"Bye, mum," I said.

"Bye, Mom" Michelle repeated in a whisper, then sniffled again.

Without looking back, we all left the bedroom. As sad as I was, I couldn't help feeling grateful that Mom would finally be set free. What happened to her was so fucked up.

CHAPTER FIFTY-FOUR

CHRIS

Letting my wife starve to death was never part of our plans for growing old together. There were so many things we were supposed to do together—travel to Montana, help our children raise our grandkids, maybe even take everyone to Disney. This wasn't one of the things I'd intended to do with my wife.

I'd tried to feed her breakfast every morning—eggs, turkey, strawberries, and coffee, but she just said, "no." Our kids tried to get her to eat, too, but after only seven days of not eating, she began to tell them that she had "already made it this far, and she wasn't turning around." After that, we all stopped trying to force the issue. There was nothing we could do to change her mind. It was okay. You know what? As much as it hurt me to see, she was finally the one in control, and I couldn't help but feel proud of her.

Everything was actually happening exactly the way she wanted. She didn't have any infections. She wouldn't die "full of shit." She wasn't going to have a heart attack. And thank G-d, she was home—the place she loved most in the entire world.

Her bed was set up right next to the window. For the past twenty months, she liked to look outside and watch the world go on around her. She kept a close eye on the comings and goings of all our neighbors, and never hesitated to text them when they left their garage door open by accident. We kept candles burning constantly on the window sill. Cinnamon and lavender were her favorite scents, so I kept them in stock at all times. I didn't want to run out of candles, but we were running out of places to put them. Every night, when I closed her window shade, I had to move all of the candles and potted plants to her dresser on the other side of the room. Then, every morning at six a.m., I'd open the shade and put everything back in its spot. Yeah, we had a good routine, my wife and I.

For the last couple of weeks, we had hospice nurses visiting around the clock. Misha, a real hot ticket whom Tammy loved,

217

came every day at nine a.m. to cleanse her skin and lather her in lotion. Laurie, her other nurse-turned-best-friend, visited in the afternoons to check her medicines and make sure she wasn't in pain. Hospice nurses don't usually get to see the same patient for twenty months straight. But these did. They loved visiting Tammy.

The weaker her body grew, the more purple haze we'd pump into her IV. We didn't want her to feel any pain. Eventually, she was so weak that you needed to lean right next to her ear to hear her barely audible words.

"Water," she'd croak, her right arm flailing around lazily in the air above her, about ten times a day.

"You want some water, baby? Okay, here you go." I'd hold the straw from her sippy cup to her lips and watch her take a tiny sip. She could only take tiny sips. We all knew she wasn't drinking enough to keep herself alive.

Every night, I slept in the chair beside her, terrified that if I slept anywhere else, I'd miss something. It was the same chair that Tammy had learned to live in as her MS progressed. The chair had become so worn-in that it barely provided any support for my aching back. It was incredibly uncomfortable, but I didn't care. I wasn't complaining. If I hadn't woken up limping every morning, no one would have ever known how much physical pain I was in. My pain paled in comparison to what my wife was going through.

During all hours of the day and night, I keep a close watch on her, monitoring her for signs of the faintest distress. Did her eyes just squeeze more tightly shut? Did she need another sip of water? Did she need her feet to be wiggled? Were her muscles sore? I could read every tiny movement and know exactly what she needed. Even her nurses would look to me for answers of how to comfort her. No one knew my baby the way I did.

I still kissed her every time I left the room, never knowing when it would be our last.

On day thirty-one of little food and water, my sister came to visit. It was a Friday morning, and rain was falling lightly outside. I had a bill I needed to pay, and I liked to pay them in person at the store. The only reason I felt okay about leaving was that

Trudy was there.

Trudy made herself comfortable in the bedroom with Tammy, whose skin had become yet another shade more translucent. Her face had shrunken in so much that you could see the outline of her skull. She hadn't even tried to speak for about two weeks. She just slept and breathed.

I walked to the kitchen and put on my boots. "Bye, Luck! Be a good dog. I'll be right back." I gave Lucky a pat on the head, then began to shut the door behind me as the garage door started to lift.

Suddenly, I heard Trudy walking toward me from the bedroom.

"Chris, something's changing. Don't leave," Trudy said, panic in her voice.

Immediately, I turned around, slammed the door shut behind me and dropped my keys onto the counter. My boots bounded on the hardwood as I began making strides toward her room like I had done so many times before when I heard her screaming for help. Except this time, there was no screaming. I never would have imagined that there would come a day when I would prefer to hear her screams instead of silence. "What's going on?" I asked her.

"I don't know . . ." Trudy responded empathetically. "I think her breathing is changing." We had always considered Trudy the angel of the family. We always thought she had a sixth sense about these things.

Trudy trailed right behind me while I strode toward our bedroom. I walked right up to the bed, where my wife of thirty-three years lay motionless, and wrapped my arms around tightly her whole body, lifting her out of her bed just slightly to get my arms behind her back. I leaned on the edge of her bed and began whispering in her ear, the tears suddenly returning.

"Tammy, baby, I love you. It's okay baby. I'll take care of the kids. I promise. It's okay." I kissed her forehead, then her lips, and kept repeating it over and over, unsure if I was reminding her or myself that I would be okay. I waited for a response, but there was none.

"It's okay," I stuttered, wiping tears with the back of my hand. I looked from Tammy to Trudy, and we both knew what was happening.

"It's okay," I said again. "You can go home now."

And just like that, she slipped away.

CHAPTER FIFTY-FIVE

TAMMY

Whenever my family took a trip, I used to say the same thing every single time we arrived, safe and sound, back at our home. As we pulled into our driveway and the garage door began to open, it didn't matter where we went or how long we were gone, I would still always say it.

Home again, home again, jiggity jig.

For years, my MS held me captive in my home. My home used to be my favorite place in the world. MS made my home the *only* place in my world. And yet, I still loved being home, even if it was the only place I had.

I loved the phrase *home again, home again, jiggity jig.* I loved the comfort that came with saying it—the moment that I realized I was returning to the place where I came from, where I would always belong.

Thanks to Chris, I was able to receive at-home hospice care for twenty months. My family and all the wonderful hospice nurses who took care of me every day enabled me to feel as comfortable and safe as possible in my own home. But I had been choking a lot lately, and I was having a hard time breathing. My hospice nurses prescribed me pain medicines so I wouldn't feel pain from the muscle spasms, which felt like shards of glass dragging through my body. I was safe. I was comfortable. My family was . . . well, together. They were cemented together more tightly than ever before. They would be okay—they had each other.

That phrase . . . *home again, home again, jiggity jig,* had been sticking with me lately. I doubted I would ever leave my home again. I knew that if I were to ever say the phrase again, even if I were already at home, my family would understand why I said it. If they were indeed the last words I said, it would, somehow, make sense.

In the literal sense, I was already home. I was surrounded by a loving family and frequent visitors. I had wonderful hospice nurses who took amazing care of me and became my best friends. But the other home, the one all eventually return to, was waiting for me.

I wouldn't be sad when I said those words for the very last time. Instead, there would be a sort of peacefulness to them.

The peace would come from knowing that I *was* stronger than MS.

I *did* beat MS.

It *didn't* beat me.

Don't believe me?

Do you need proof?

Just look at the family I created. Just look at the life that I lived.

*_*_*_*_*_*

Home again, home again, jiggity jig.

EPILOGUE
MICHELLE

I used to think that there was no such thing as *fighting* MS. I used to think that no matter how hard Mom tried to fight it, MS was going to beat her. And maybe, had Dad been anyone else, that might have been true. But because of him, and the way he stood by our family every single day, no matter what MS threw at us, in the end, we did win. Because, above all else, he showed us how to stick together.

Her obituary said that she died from complications of her MS. And I suppose, in the very literal sense, that was true. Her inability to move, swallow, and breathe were indeed what killed her on that rainy morning in August while Dad held her tightly in his arms, eight months after she first considered swallowing the pills. But her MS did not win at the game of stealing her life, and it will not win at claiming her death either. Her insurmountable strength won. Her positivity won. Her attitude and outlook on all things in her life won. *She won.*

~~*~*~*~*

Knowing someone who has MS makes it so easy to grieve for all that is lost along the way, to focus on everything that used to be, to wish for all the things that had been ripped from your lives to be given back to you. MS doesn't make it easy to appreciate the remaining shreds of what life *used to be*. It's not easy to think about what that person who you love still has left. What MS hasn't taken yet. The things they can still do.

If you know someone with a chronic illness like MS, you won't notice anything changing as each day passes. You won't notice the subtle loss of function as it drifts steadily away. But, once one, two, or ten years have gone by, you'll look back and realize there was something that person you love used to be able to do that they can't anymore.

Appreciate everything they still have. Cherish those shopping trips and late-night conversations. Laugh when things get dropped all over the floor at Rite Aid. Don't be upset when the cane turns into a walker. Just be glad they're still moving. Smile when things get hard. And remember that they could be *so* much harder.

I'm not saying you should be happy and grateful *every day.* Actually, I'm saying the opposite—I'm saying it's okay to feel sad sometimes. Just don't be so busy feeling sad that you forget to see everything you still have left. I know that sometimes it's really hard to see what's left. But I promise it is there . . . you just have to be willing to take another look.

~~*~*~*~*

I'd love to know why you read this book. I am a person who reads for enjoyment, to pass the time, to be transported out of my own life into the world of someone else's. I like to read stories that inspire me to be a better person, to live life slightly differently than before. I like to know what it feels like to walk in the shoes of people whom I know I will never be, whose lives I would never lead myself.

I wonder if you picked up this book because you know someone who is fighting an invisible battle. Maybe it's you. Maybe it's your daughter, son, aunt, uncle, niece, or nephew. Maybe it's your mom or dad. Maybe you wanted to understand what was really going through their mind when you asked how they were doing, and they said "good," but you swore you saw a flicker of pain in their eyes. And you wanted to push to find out more, but you didn't know how. If so, then now you know the truth. At least, you know mine.

Maybe you just wanted to learn about MS because you or someone you love has been diagnosed. If so, please remember that every case of MS is extremely different. My mom's story is not *your* story. But at the very least, I hope you know that you aren't the only one who hates MS.

Were you scared to read this story? Were you as scared to read this as Mom was to read about Annette Funicello? If you were, it's okay. To be honest, I was a little scared to write it all down. And I'm pretty sure Mom was scared to live it.

How's Your Mom?

Right now, I don't know what the lesson is from this journey that G-d put my family on with the villain that tried to steal our lives. Perhaps time will tell. For now, for whatever reason you read this book, I hope you know one thing—you are not alone.

There are others who are fighting invisible battles, and who want to listen to the truth. You don't always have to say that everything is "good." Sometimes life isn't good. Sometimes you need to feel the pain. Talking to someone about it won't always make everything better. But it helps to know you're not alone.

And if you can't speak about things out loud, you can always try writing them down in a book. Maybe, say, a twelve-dollar one with yellow and orange flowers?

ACKNOWLEDGEMENTS

Thank you to my mom, who is now a dragonfly always watching over us. Thank you for loving and supporting me through all of the seasons of my life. I was incredibly lucky to have you as my mom. I miss you every day.

This book wouldn't have been possible without the constant support and love of my husband, Tyler. Thank you for all times you let me talk your ear off and for always encouraging me to write down my family's story. Thank you for letting me read you chapters out loud and completely monopolize date nights by talking about this book. Thank you for letting me tell you the truth when you asked how I was doing, and for continuing to ask the question even when you thought you knew the answer. You are the best thing that has ever happened to me.

Thank you to all of my family and friends who have continuously supported me and listened to me while I've talked on and on about this book. I couldn't have done it without you all.

Thank you to my editor, Rebecca Mahoney, who inadvertently became my therapist and mentor while we worked through several iterations of this story. Thank you, Rebecca, for believing in me and seeing the light that was buried beneath the darkness.

Thank you Ardra Shepard, my favorite MS Blogger (*Tripping on Air*) for writing so honestly about MS and allowing me to feel like it was okay to do the same. Thank you for being one of the first people to read this story and encouraging me to publish it. Together, we just might change the public's awareness of Progressive MS.

CPSIA information can be obtained
at www.ICGtesting.com
Printed in the USA
BVHW06s0937221018
530870BV00031B/2035/P